THE JOHNS HOPKINS
Manual for GI Endoscopic Nurses
Third Edition

Manual for GI Endoscopic Nurses
Third Edition

Editors

Mouen A. Khashab, MD

Toshunia F. Robinson, RN, BSN

Anthony N. Kalloo, MD

Johns Hopkins University
Department of Gastroenterology
Baltimore, Maryland

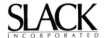

www.Healio.com/books

ISBN: 978-1-61711-051-1

Copyright © 2014 by SLACK Incorporated

The previous edition of *Johns Hopkins Manual of Gastrointestinal Endoscopic Procedures, Second Edition* was written by Dr. Anthony Kalloo, MD along with Jeanette Ogilvie, RN, BSN, CGRN and Lisa M. Hicks, RN, BSN, CGRN

The procedures and practices described in this publication should be implemented in a manner consistent with the professional standards set for the circumstances that apply in each specific situation. Every effort has been made to confirm the accuracy of the information presented and to correctly relate generally accepted practices. The authors, editors, and publisher cannot accept responsibility for errors or exclusions or for the outcome of the material presented herein. There is no expressed or implied warranty of this book or information imparted by it. Care has been taken to ensure that drug selection and dosages are in accordance with currently accepted/recommended practice. Off-label uses of drugs may be discussed. Due to continuing research, changes in government policy and regulations, and various effects of drug reactions and interactions, it is recommended that the reader carefully review all materials and literature provided for each drug, especially those that are new or not frequently used. Some drugs or devices in this publication have clearance for use in a restricted research setting by the Food and Drug and Administration or FDA. Each professional should determine the FDA status of any drug or device prior to use in their practice.

Any review or mention of specific companies or products is not intended as an endorsement by the author or publisher.

SLACK Incorporated uses a review process to evaluate submitted material. Prior to publication, educators or clinicians provide important feedback on the content that we publish. We welcome feedback on this work.

Published by: SLACK Incorporated
                     6900 Grove Road
                     Thorofare, NJ 08086 USA
                     Telephone: 856-848-1000
                     Fax: 856-848-6091
                     www.Healio.com/books

Contact SLACK Incorporated for more information about other books in this field or about the availability of our books from distributors outside the United States.

Library of Congress Cataloging-in-Publication Data
Khashab, Mouen, author.
 The John Hopkins manual for GI endoscopic nurses / Mouen Khashab, Toshunia Robinson, Anthony Kalloo. -- Third edition.
  p. ; cm.
 Manual for GI endoscopic nurses
 Preceded by: Johns Hopkins manual of gastrointestinal endoscopy procedures / Jeanette Ogilvie, Lisa M. Hicks, Anthony N. Kalloo. 2nd ed. c2008.
 Includes bibliographical references and index.
 ISBN 978-1-61711-051-1 (alk. paper)
 I. Robinson, Toshunia, author. II. Kalloo, Anthony, 1955- author. III. Ogilvie, Jeanette, 1949- Johns Hopkins manual of gastrointestinal endoscopy procedures. Preceded by (work): IV. Title. V. Title: Manual for GI endoscopic nurses.
 [DNLM: 1. Endoscopy, Gastrointestinal--nursing--Handbooks. 2. Endoscopy, Gastrointestinal--methods--Handbooks. 3. Gastrointestinal Diseases--nursing--Handbooks. WY 49]
 RC804.E6
 616.3'307545--dc23
                          2013025715
For permission to reprint material in another publication, contact SLACK Incorporated. Authorization to photocopy items for internal, personal, or academic use is granted by SLACK Incorporated provided that the appropriate fee is paid directly to Copyright Clearance Center. Prior to photocopying items, please contact the Copyright Clearance Center at 222 Rosewood Drive, Danvers, MA 01923 USA; phone: 978-750-8400; website: www.copyright.com; email: info@copyright.com

Printed in the United States of America.

Last digit is print number: 10   9   8   7   6   5   4   3

DEDICATION

This manual is dedicated to the hard-working and devoted physicians, nurses, and nursing assistants of the endoscopy units at Johns Hopkins Hospital.

CONTENTS

Contents

Contents

Contents

Contents

Acknowledgments

The current editors would like to acknowledge the immense contributions of the editors of the previous (second) edition of the manual, Jeanette Ogilvie and Lisa M. Hicks. Also, we would like to acknowledge the artistic contributions of Michael S. Linkinhoker, MA, CMI, for his medical illustrations and photography. The medical illustrations were reproduced courtesy of the Johns Hopkins Gastroenterology and Hepatology Web site at www. hopkins-gi.org.

ABOUT THE EDITORS

Mouen A. Khashab, MD is an assistant professor of medicine at the Johns Hopkins University School of Medicine and director of therapeutic endoscopy at Johns Hopkins Hospital. He is an expert on various aspects of therapeutic endoscopy and endoscopy innovations and is well-published in the field.

Toshunia F. Robinson, RN, BSN has been a medical/surgical nurse for over 13 years. Currently she is a clinical nurse educator at Johns Hopkins Hospital Endoscopy Unit. She is an expert in diagnostic and therapeutic endoscopy procedures and has presented at several regional conferences.

Anthony N. Kalloo, MD is a professor of medicine at the Johns Hopkins University School of Medicine. He is currently Chief of Gastroenterology and Hepatology at the Johns Hopkins University School of Medicine. Dr. Kalloo has a national and international reputation as a therapeutic endoscopist and an innovative researcher.

CONTRIBUTING AUTHORS

Gerard Aguila, RN, BSN
Department of Endoscopy
Johns Hopkins Hospital
Baltimore, Maryland

Stuart K. Amateau, MD, PhD
Assistant Professor of Medicine
Director of Bariatric Endoscopy and Tissue Apposition
Therapeutic and Interventional Endoscopy
Division of Gastroenterology and Hepatology
University of Colorado Anschutz Medical Campus
Aurora, Colorado

Rukshana Cader, MD
Gastroenterologist
Trinity Health
Minot, North Dakota

Marcia Irene Canto, MD, MHS
Professor of Medicine
Johns Hopkins University School of Medicine
Department of Medicine, Division of Gastroenterology and Hepatology
Baltimore, Maryland

Victor Chedid, MD
Postdoctoral Research Fellow
Division of Gastroenterology & Hepatology
Johns Hopkins University School of Medicine
Baltimore, Maryland

John Clarke, MD
Assistant Professor of Medicine
Division of Gastroenterology & Hepatology
Johns Hopkins University School of Medicine
Baltimore, Maryland

Contributing Authors

Sameer Dhalla, MD, MHS
Assistant Professor of Medicine
Division of Gastroenterology and Hepatology
Johns Hopkins University School of Medicine
Baltimore, Maryland

Rosa Maria Fusco, RN, BSN, CGRN
Clinical Nurse
Department of Endoscopy
Johns Hopkins Hospital
Baltimore, Maryland

Eduardo Gonzalez-Velez, MD
Assistant Professor of Gastroenterology
Johns Hopkins Hospital
Baltimore, Maryland

Claudia Guilbeau-Brand, RN, MSN, CGRN
Clinical Nurse Endoscopy / Clinical Instructor
Division of Gastroenterology
Johns Hopkins Hospital/ Johns Hopkins University School of Nursing

Christina Ha, MD
Johns Hopkins School of Medicine
Assistant Professor
Division of Gastroenterology and Hepatology
Baltimore, Maryland

Anne Marie Lennon, MD
Assistant Professor of Medicine,
Department of Gastroenterology,
Johns Hopkins Medical Institutions
Baltimore, Maryland

Zhiping Li, MD
Associate Professor of Medicine
Director of Hepatology
Johns Hopkins University
Baltimore, Maryland

Contributing Authors

Libbie L. Monroe, RN, BSN, CGRN
Department of Gastroenterology and Hepatology
Johns Hopkins Hospital
Baltimore, Maryland

Lisette Musaib-Ali, MD
Internist
Jai Medical Center
Baltimore, Maryland

Patrick I. Okolo III, MD, MPH
Associate Professor of Medicine
Chief of Endoscopy
Johns Hopkins Hospital
Baltimore, Maryland

Reem Sharaiha, MD, MSc
Assistant Professor of Medicine
Advanced Endoscopy
Division of Gastroenterology & Hepatology
Department of Medicine
Weill Cornell Medical College
New York, New York

Eun Ji Shin, MD
Assistant Professor of Medicine
Co-Director of the Gastroenterology Fellowship program
Director of Advanced Endoscopy Fellowship Program
Johns Hopkins Hospital
Division of Gastroenterology and Hepatology
Baltimore, Maryland

Vikesh K. Singh, MD, MSc
Assistant Professor of Medicine
Director, Pancreatitis Center
Medical Director, Pancreatic Islet Autotransplantation Program
Division of Gastroenterology
Johns Hopkins Hospital
Baltimore, Maryland

Contributing Authors

Ellen Stein, MD
Assistant Professor of Medicine
Division of Gastroenterology & Hepatology
Johns Hopkins Hospital
Baltimore, Maryland

David W. Victor III, MD
Instructor of Medicine
Johns Hopkins Hospital
Division of Gastroenterology and Hepatology
Baltimore, Maryland

Janet Yoder, RN, CGRN
Nurse Clinician III
Department of Medicine Endoscopy
Johns Hopkins Hospital
Baltimore, Maryland

FOREWORD

I am delighted to have been invited to contribute a few words to this magnificent book, a comprehensive guide to optimizing outcomes for patients undergoing the whole range of endoscopic procedures.

Some of us can remember (well one of us, anyway) the days when endoscopy (actually then only gastroscopy) was an occasional adventure carried out in the side room of a ward with a passing nurse to assist.

My first "endoscopy unit" was a converted wet lab in a research area called the "Gut Hut" at St. Thomas's hospital in London.

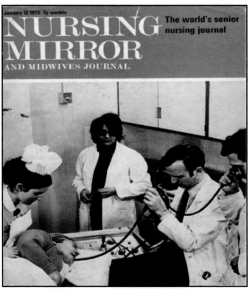

Reprinted with permission from EMAP Publishing Limited Company.

The picture shows the scene in 1972, with my first official endoscopy nurse, Sue Wright, in her Florence Nightingale uniform, and a bored chemistry tech holding biopsy forceps. There was a small curtained area in the corridor for "recovery."

We have all come a long way since then (including using gloves!).

Over the last 40 years it has been my privilege to organize endoscopy units of increasing complexity and size at The Middlesex Hospital in London, Duke University Medical Center in Durham, North Carolina,

Foreword

and at the Medical University of South Carolina. The early occasional pioneering adventures have morphed into a sophisticated business.

Digestive endoscopy is very much a team event, at every level, from small office units to major referral centers. It requires solid leadership and educated and dedicated staff with a wide variety of skill sets.

I have been deeply fortunate in recent years to have worked with superb teams, and two outstanding nurse-managers, Marilyn Schaffner and Phyllis Malpas. Both have been Presidents of the American Society for Gastrointestinal Nurses and Assistants (SGNA). Phyllis now manages no fewer than 35 endoscopy nurses, 12 technical specialists, 3 patient care technicians, and some administrative personnel. Each member of the team knows his or her role and respects those of others.

An endoscopy unit now functions like a large symphony orchestra, with a variety of well-trained professionals working in unison to produce wonderful results. But, like any orchestra, one person playing out of tune can ruin everything.

I congratulate the authors and contributors to this book for providing the latest sheet music with which the endoscopy team can combine to produce concerts of the highest quality.

And I salute those who use this resource to enhance their services, not least those in the "back corridor" (eg, the reprocessing staff) whose work is so important but rarely celebrated. Thank you all.

Peter B. Cotton, MD
Professor of Medicine
Medical University of South Carolina
Charleston, South Carolina

INTRODUCTION

This manual is intended as a quick reference for users of the gastrointestinal endoscopy unit. It should be especially helpful for nurses who have the responsibility of preparing patients for endoscopic procedures. It provides endoscopic preparation regimens to facilitate the correct instruction of patients, reducing the likelihood of unsuccessful procedures. This manual should be regarded as a reference; deference should always be given to the patients' physician preferences.

We have provided the definitions and indications for common endoscopic procedures along with listings of necessary equipment. Chapters that appeared in the previous edition are updated and multiple new chapters have been added. These new chapters are meant to render the book more comprehensive and to cover common, less common, and new endoscopic procedures. We have used photographs and illustrations in place of detailed descriptions. (Individual employers should provide in-service training on all equipment being utilized by employees in their facility.) Nursing care before, during, and after endoscopic procedures is outlined. Finally, general guidelines for moderate sedation and equipment disinfection and sterilization are discussed, as well as antibiotic coverage and special considerations for patients with specific medical conditions who are undergoing endoscopy.

Chapter 1

THE CHANGING WORLD OF GASTROINTESTINAL ENDOSCOPY

Libbie L. Monroe, BSN, RN, CGRN AND
Toshunia F. Robinson, RN, BSN

The beginnings of endoscopy are said to have taken place when Adolph Kussmaul placed a rigid tube into the stomach of a professional sword swallower in 1868. Rudolph Schindler, who is called the "father of endoscopy," published the first textbook on gastroscopy in 1923. The first colonoscopy was performed in 1955 and 2 years later, fiberoptic endoscopy was introduced. In the third quarter of the 20th century, gastrointestinal endoscopy was considered to be a diagnostic modality. However, the performance of the first polypectomy in 1971 by Doctors Wolff and Shinya probably heralded the field of therapeutic endoscopy. Their findings were ultimately published in a paper in the *New England Journal of Medicine* in 1973.

The timeline of these historic endoscopic milestones illustrates the relatively short history of gastrointestinal endoscopy. It is amazing to think that the first experience of colonoscopy with a videoendoscope was published by Doctors Sivak and Fleischer in 1984. Gastrointestinal endoscopists and gastrointestinal assistants are now faced with a bewildering array of diagnostic and interventional procedures that are rapidly evolving. It is becoming more challenging for endoscopy mangers to handle endoscopic supplies and plan for procedures with the wide portfolio of endoscopic procedures and accessories.

The word *endoscopy* is derived from the Greek word *endo,* which means "within," and *scopein,* which means "to look." Our ability "to look within" and formulate diagnoses have evolved dramatically in the last few years, even since the last edition of this manual. Old chapters have

Khashab MA, Robinson TF, Kalloo AN.
The Johns Hopkins Manual for GI Endoscopic Nurses,
Third Edition (pp 1-2).
© 2014 SLACK Incorporated.

been updated to include recent advances in the field. In addition, there has been a recent leap into minimally invasive approaches for treatment and/or palliation of gastrointestinal and pancreaticobiliary diseases. As a result, new sections have been added to this manual to give you a glimpse of the future with regards to diagnostic and therapeutic modalities.

We have seen a significant increase in the use of cholangioscopy for the diagnosis and treatment of different biliary disorders in the last few years. As a result, a new section on single-operator cholangioscopy has been added to the new edition (p.154). Other recent therapeutic advances include endoscopic-ultrasonography-guided fiducial placement for image-guided high-dose radiation therapy for pancreatic cancer. A dedicated section describing set-up and techniques used is now included (p.104). Similarly, the use of radiofrequency ablation for the treatment of Barrett's esophagus and associated dysplasia has boomed, as level I evidence is now available for its effectiveness and safety. Details of this technique are now described in a dedicated section (p.63). Other new sections include endoscopic therapy of achalasia, foreign body retrieval, impedance-PH testing, and others.

As in the previous two editions, this updated manual will serve to provide you with a quick but comprehensive set-up and how-to technique for most gastrointestinal endoscopy procedures. The future of gastrointestinal endoscopy is bright both from a diagnostic and therapeutic standpoint. We hope that this manual will serve to simplify this rapidly evolving field, and in the process improve the lives of our patients.

Chapter 2

ROLE OF THE ENDOSCOPY NURSE

*LIBBIE L. MONROE, RN, BSN, CGRN AND
TOSHUNIA F. ROBINSON, RN, BSN*

Nurse-administered sedation is integral to endoscopy practice. Historically, the nurse had more patient care responsibilities while working in the procedure rooms. It was not unusual for the nurse to assist the physician with the procedure, while at the same time administering sedation and monitoring vital signs. This is not a feasible practice anymore due to an increase in procedural complexity and the number of comorbid patients. Two nurses are frequently needed to work in therapeutic rooms, even when an anesthesia provider is caring for the patient. This practice is an absolute requirement when the nurse is administering conscious sedation. Nontherapeutic rooms can be staffed by a nurse and a clinical technician.

In the past, the majority of sedation was performed by registered nurses and it was acceptable to have a 3:1 nurse-to-patient ratio following conscious sedation. However, with the initiation of monitored sedation administered by anesthesia providers, it has become necessary to have nurses receive post anesthesia care unit (PACU) training/certification. In addition, the optimal nurse-to-patient ratio has become 2:1 in such practices.

The current role of the endoscopy nurse has evolved to more of a technical support function in units that implement monitored anesthesia care. Nonetheless, many units continue to employ nurse-administered sedation, often due to cost reasons. Sedation competencies must be maintained annually. As the nurse's focus has moved more toward electronic documentation and assisting physicians with complicated

Khashab MA, Robinson TF, Kalloo AN.
*The Johns Hopkins Manual for GI Endoscopic Nurses,
Third Edition* (pp 3-4).
© 2014 SLACK Incorporated.

Chapter 2

procedures, it has become increasingly more evident that continuing education and hands-on practice with endoscopic equipment and accessories need to be addressed at routine intervals.

Chapter 3

Intravenous Moderate Sedation Guidelines

Claudia Guilbeau-Brand, RN, MSN, CGRN

Intravenous Conscious Sedation

The delivery of health care in the field of gastroenterology has become more complex and diversified. The days of physician-administered sedation and a nurse and/or technician assisting with little or no patient monitoring are gone. Today, the registered nurse (RN) administers moderate sedation (previously referred to as conscious sedation) assisted by a plethora of monitoring devices. Most gastrointestinal (GI) units staff a physician, RN, and technician in the room. In some instances there are two nurses in attendance.

The Society of Gastrointestinal Nurses and Associates, Inc (SGNA) has outlined a position statement regarding the administration of intravenous moderate sedation to patients undergoing endoscopy. While this position statement provides an appropriate guideline for moderate sedation, it is important for the nurse to follow the guidelines of his or her own state board of nursing and hospital accreditation agency. The SGNA statement maintains that RNs trained and experienced in gastroenterology nursing and endoscopy be given the responsibility of administration and maintenance of sedation and analgesia by order of a physician. The RN is responsible for the administration of reversal agents also prescribed by the physician.

Khashab MA, Robinson TF, Kalloo AN.
The Johns Hopkins Manual for GI Endoscopic Nurses,
Third Edition (pp 5-14).
© 2014 SLACK Incorporated.

Chapter 3

The nurse must be knowledgeable about the pharmacology of drugs used for sedation; their indications, contraindications, mechanism of actions; as well as drugs used to reverse their actions. Additionally, the RN must have the knowledge and skills needed to assess, diagnose, and intervene in case of complications.

The SGNA recommends that two RNs or one RN and a trained associate be present with the physician in each procedure room to handle the equipment proficiently. During endoscopic procedures, the nurse provides sedation and monitors the patient while an associate assists with the procedure.

AMERICAN SOCIETY OF ANESTHESIOLOGISTS CLASSIFICATION

The American Society of Anesthesiologists (ASA) classification is useful in characterizing a patient's ability to tolerate sedation, anesthesia, and stress. Physicians should use this six-step classification to determine if moderate sedation can be accomplished without causing harm to the patient:

- Class I: The patient is healthy and has no underlying organic disease. This is the typical patient seen in an outpatient or free-standing endoscopy center for a diagnostic esophagogastroduodenoscopy (EGD) or colonoscopy.
- Class II: The patient has mild-to-moderate systemic disease that does not interfere with daily routines. Examples: hypertension with a history of coronary artery bypass graft surgery without symptoms; well-controlled asthma, anemia, or diabetes; age older than 70 years; and pregnancy.
- Class III: Severe systemic disturbance such as diseases from any cause, poorly controlled hypertension, poorly controlled diabetes mellitus, symptomatic respiratory disease, such as asthma or chronic obstructive pulmonary disease, and massive obesity.
- Class IV: Life-threatening severe systemic disorders such as unstable angina, debilitating respiratory disease, and end-stage renal disease.
- Class V: Moribund with little chance of survival.
- Class VI: Emergent; any patient who must undergo emergent endoscopy.

DEFINITION OF MODERATE SEDATION

Moderate sedation and analgesia refers to the drug-induced state that allows the patient to tolerate unpleasant sensations while still maintaining control of protective reflexes. The ability to respond purposefully to tactile and verbal stimulation is within the patient's control.

PRINCIPLES OF MODERATE SEDATION

The following principles of moderate sedation should be followed in all settings when performing endoscopy.

PREPROCEDURE

- Individuals responsible for delivering moderate sedation and patient assessment should be trained in basic cardiac life support.
- It is recommended that a person with advanced cardiac life support training be accessible and on the premises.
- The nurse administering sedation and analgesia should be familiar with all medication actions, dosages, recommendations for titration, side effects, and reversal medications.
- Competency for administration of analgesia and sedation should be a part of orientation for all those who administer moderate sedation. The following is a list of the current criteria:
  1. Demonstrate acquired knowledge of anatomy, physiology, pharmacology, and complications related to intravenous sedation and analgesia.
  2. Demonstrate assessment skills during intravenous sedation, analgesia, and recovery.
  3. Understand the principles of oxygen delivery, respiratory physiology, transport, and uptake.
  4. Demonstrate proficiency in airway management, including the ability to use oxygen-delivery devices.
  5. Have knowledge of potential complications of intravenous sedation and analgesia in relation to the type of medication administered.
  6. Demonstrate skills to assess, diagnose, and intervene in situations consistent with institutional protocols and guidelines.
  7. Be knowledgeable regarding age-specific needs of patient populations under the staff members' care.

Chapter 3

INTRAPROCEDURE

- Throughout the procedure, verbal reassurance should be provided to the patient. This may improve patient tolerance and decrease the sedation required.
- Continued patient assessment and monitoring of physiologic parameters (eg, vital signs, cardiac rhythm, and oxygen saturation), level of comfort, warmth and dryness of skin, and level of consciousness.
- Vital signs should be documented at baseline and at least every 2 minutes during the initial sedation. After administration of the initial sedation, vital signs should be documented at 15-minute intervals unless the patient's condition warrants more frequent monitoring.
- Reversal medications should be readily available but not routinely administered.
- An emergency cart must be immediately accessible where moderate (conscious) sedation is being administered.

POSTPROCEDURE

- Monitoring may be discontinued when the patient's vital signs return to baseline or other criteria established by the individual institution.

DEFINITION OF DEEP SEDATION

Deep sedation and analgesia refers to the drug-induced depression of consciousness during which sedatives or a combination of sedatives and analgesic medications and/or anesthetizing agents are administered. Deep sedation limits the ability of the patient to maintain protective reflexes (ie, airway, breathing, coughing). The ability to respond to verbal and tactile stimuli is compromised.

PRINCIPLES OF DEEP SEDATION

The following principles of deep sedation should be followed in all settings when performing endoscopy. Since sedation exists along a continuum, deep sedation may be an unplanned outcome of moderate sedation. Planned deep sedation should only be administered by persons trained in the administration of general anesthesia.

PREPROCEDURE

- Same as for moderate sedation.

INTRAPROCEDURE

- Same as for moderate sedation.

POSTPROCEDURE

- Same as for moderate sedation

ACTIONS, DOSAGES, AND SIDE EFFECTS OF COMMONLY USED INTRAVENOUS MODERATE SEDATION DRUGS

In general, the drugs used for moderate sedation and analgesia routinely consist of a combination of a narcotic such as fentanyl (a short-acting synthetic narcotic) or meperidine (a longer-acting narcotic) and a tranquilizer such as midazolam or diazepam. Other benzodiazepines may be substituted depending upon the preference of the institution or physician.

In patients who are refractory to sedation, the physician may request administration of other drugs to potentiate the action of the narcotic, such as promethazine hydrochloride, which is a phenothiazine, or a butyrophenone such as droperidol.

FENTANYL

Short-acting synthetic narcotic used to produce sedation or analgesia in patients receiving endoscopy. Fentanyl binds with opiate receptors in the central nervous system, altering both emotional and perceptual response to pain.

- Dosage: 25 to 75 mcg slowly over 2 minutes, may repeat after 3 to 4 minutes up to 3 mcg/kg
- Onset of action: Immediate
- Peak action: 1 to 3 minutes
- Duration of action: 30 to 60 minutes
- Side effects: Respiratory depression, apnea, arrest, hypotension, changes in heart rate, dizziness, circulatory collapse or arrest, nausea, vomiting, and constipation
- Antagonist: Naloxone (Narcan)

Chapter 3

Meperidine

Longer-acting opioid used to produce sedation or analgesia. Same action on the central nervous system as fentanyl.

- Dosage: 25 to 50 mg over 1 to 2 minutes, repeat after 2 to 3 minutes as needed
- Onset of action: 3 to 5 minutes
- Peak action: 30 to 60 minutes
- Duration of action: 2 to 4 hours
- Side effects: Same as for fentanyl
- Antagonist: Naloxone (Narcan)

Midazolam

Benzodiazepine depresses the central nervous system at limbic and subcortical levels of the brain. Produces sedative effect and skeletal and muscular relaxation, relieves anxiety, and produces retrograde amnesia. Used in intravenous moderate sedation in combination with fentanyl or meperidine.

- Dosage: 0.03 mg/kg IV over at least 2 minutes. Do not exceed initial dose of 1.5 mg for patients over 60 years of age or 2.5 mg for patients under 60. May repeat 0.5 to 1 mg doses after 2 to 3 minutes. Usually do not exceed 5 mg total, except in cases of extended duration.
- You may continue to titrate to higher doses if needed to obtain effect. Wait at least 2 minutes after each administration of medication to determine its effect.
- Onset of action: 1 to 5 minutes.
- Peak action: 5 minutes, gradually declining over 30 to 40 minutes.
- Duration of action: Less than 2 hours. If used in combination with protease inhibitors, the half life of the drug is doubled.
- Side effects: Antegrade amnesia, lethargy or excessive drowsiness, respiratory depression, airway obstruction, laryngospasms, light-headedness, hypotension, tachycardia, and cardiovascular collapse
- Antagonist: Flumazenil

Diazepam

A benzodiazepine; same action as midazolam.

- Dosage: Titrate 1 to 5 mg until desired effect achieved; 5 mg end-point for elderly and debilitated, 10 mg endpoint for healthy adult.
- Onset of action: 1 to 3 minutes
- Peak action: 15 to 30 minutes
- Duration of action: 2 to 4 hours

- Side effects: Same as midazolam
- Antagonist: Flumazenil

DROPERIDOL

A butyrophenone; acts primarily in the central nervous system at the subcortical level to cause sedation and decrease the incidence of nausea and vomiting. No analgesic effects.

- Dosage: Initial dose 1.25 to 2.5 mg over 2 minutes. Repeat doses of 0.625 to 1.25 mg may be given after 5 minutes of initial dose. Maximum dose is 6 to 10 mg.
- Onset of action: 3 to 10 minutes, wait at least 5 minutes to assess full effect
- Peak action: 10 to 30 minutes
- Duration of action: 2 to 4 hours
- Side effects: Hypotension, tachycardia, dizziness, drowsiness, dystonic reactions, Parkinsonian signs and symptoms, severe hypotension leading to cardiovascular collapse; alteration of consciousness may last up to 12 hours. Should be used with extreme caution in patients with risk factors for prolonged Q-T syndrome, concomitant use of antiarrhythmics, MAO inhibitors, erythromycin, haloperidol; age > 65 years; or alcohol abuse.

PROMETHAZINE

A phenothiazine, promethazine provides clinically useful sedative, antiemetic, and anticholinergic effects. Used in combination with narcotics to promote a sedative effect, it is possible to achieve optimal sedation with doses of 6.25 to 12.5 mg. Recommend diluting 25 mg vial in 20 cc normal saline and injecting in the most distal IV port to lessen the burning at the infusion site.

- Dosage: 25 to 50 mg in combination with reduced dosages of narcotics
- Onset of action: 3 to 10 minutes
- Peak action: 30 minutes
- Duration of action: 75 minutes, but effects of the drug may last 2 to 4 hours
- Side effects: Drowsiness, extrapyramidal reactions, tachycardia, bradycardia, venous thrombosis at injection site, hives, and asthma

Chapter 3

Naloxone

Narcotic analgesic antagonist used to reverse the effects of opioids during IV moderate sedation.

- Dosage: 0.1 to 0.2 mg every 2 to 3 minutes until the patient responds. Must be administered in incremental doses in order to evaluate patient response. May be delivered via any route if intravenous access is not available. Lower doses should be used in patients taking opioids chronically and in patients being treated for chronic pain.
- Onset of action: 1 to 2 minutes
- Peak action: 1 to 2 minutes
- Duration of action: 30 to 40 minutes
- Side effects: Reversal of analgesia, nausea, tachycardia, cardiac arrest, and severe hypertension if not administered in small, incremental doses. Abrupt reversal of narcotic depression can result in nausea, vomiting, sweating, tremulousness, seizures, and cardiac arrest. Narcotic abstinence symptoms induced by naloxone start to diminish in 20 to 40 minutes and disappear in 90 minutes. Not effective against barbiturates and sedatives.

Flumazenil

Benzodiazepine antagonist; competes for benzodiazepine receptor sites.

- Dosage: 0.2 mg over 15 seconds, repeat at 1-minute intervals up to 1 mg. May be repeated in 30- to 60-minute intervals to prevent resedation.
- Onset of action: 1 to 2 minutes
- Peak action: 6 to 10 minutes
- Duration of action: Frequently shorter than that of benzodiazepines. Related to the plasma levels of the benzodiazepine and the dose of flumazenil.
- Side effects: Seizures, agitation, dizziness, blurred vision, headache, increased sweating, and arrhythmias
- Monitor for a minimum of 2 hours after administration to watch for resedation. The action of flumazenil is shorter than that of benzodiazepines and does not reverse the amnesic effect of benzodiazepines.

PROPOFOL

Propofol belongs to a class of alkylphenols, sedative/hypnotic, used intravenously for the induction and maintenance of monitored anesthesia care (MAC) sedation during diagnostic procedures in adults. Propofol should be administered only by persons trained in the administration of general anesthesia. Persons administering propofol may not be involved in the endoscopic procedure.

- Dosage: Initial dose is 20 to 40 mg, followed by 10 to 20 mg boluses to maintain level of sedation
- Onset of action: 30 to 60 seconds
- Duration of action: 6 to 10 minutes, with a half-life of 1.3 to 4.13 minutes
- Side effects: Pain at injection site, hypotension, bradycardia (possible during infusion) and apnea (possible during induction)

ONDANSETRON HCL DIHYDRATE

Selective serotonin receptor antagonist, antiemetic, used for the control of pre-and postprocedure nausea and vomiting.

- Dosage: For the treatment of postoperative nausea and vomiting, a single 4-mg dose by intramuscular or slow intravenous injection (over 2 to 5 minutes) is recommended.
- Onset of action: 10 minutes
- Side effects: Headache; constipation; and the sensation of flushing or warmth, pain, redness, and burning at injection site

DOLASETRON MESYLATE

Selective serotonin receptor antagonist, antiemetic, used for the control of pre-and postprocedure nausea and vomiting.

- Dosage: 12.5 mg IV at onset of nausea and vomiting
- Onset of action: 10 minutes
- Side effects: Malaise, itching, drowsiness, chest pain, and hypotension

THE REGISTERED NURSE MANAGING AND MONITORING THE CARE OF PATIENTS RECEIVING MODERATE (CONSCIOUS) SEDATION

1. Has training beyond basic nursing preparation in the administration of moderate (conscious) sedation medications and complications

Chapter 3

related to moderate (conscious) sedation by demonstrating the following:

A. An understanding of the pharmacology of different sedation agents, their synergy, potential interactions, and adverse reactions with other medications.

B. A mastery of the titration of these agents for the desired level of sedation.

2. Demonstrates the acquired knowledge of anatomy, physiology, and cardiac arrhythmia recognition of the following:

A. Conditions associated with an increased risk of pulmonary aspiration including active upper GI hemorrhage, achalasia, bowel obstruction with gastric distension, and delayed gastric emptying.

B. Common atrial and ventricular arrhythmias, interpretation of the significance, and management of arrhythmias.

3. Assesses the total patient care requirements before and during the administration of moderate (conscious) sedation, and in the recovery phase by being able to do the following:

A. State the necessary monitoring requirements for a patient undergoing procedural sedation.

B. Demonstrate the proper use of monitoring tools during sedation: noninvasive blood pressure devices, pulse oximetry, electrocardiographic monitoring, and capnography.

C. Perform and discern the required documentation of vital signs and monitoring.

D. Identify and document the sedation scale used during the procedure.

4. Understands the principles of oxygen delivery, transport and uptake, respiratory physiology, and the use of oxygen delivery services by understanding the following:

A. Patient positioning to reduce the risk of aspiration such as elevation of the head.

B. Clinical signs of apnea and airway obstruction.

C. Indications for and use of position change and fluid bolus for management of hypotension.

5. Has the ability to intervene based upon orders or institutional protocols, in the event of complications.

6. Demonstrates competency in airway management and resuscitation (such as ACLS or PALS) appropriate to the age of the patient.

Chapter 4

CLEANING AND DISINFECTING ENDOSCOPY EQUIPMENT

JANET YODER, RN, CGRN

The proper cleaning and high-level disinfection of endoscopes and sterilization of accessory equipment are paramount in preventing transmission of infection. Standards for infection control regarding reprocessing endoscopes and endoscopic equipment have been revised over the past few years. Proper cleaning of equipment must be followed according to the manufacturer's recommendations to ensure that thorough cleaning/decontamination occurs. The following components are necessary for proper disinfection/sterilization of endoscopes and accessory equipment.

1. *Education and training:* Adherence to the principles of infection control is necessary to maintain a safe environment for patients and endoscopy personnel.

   A. Standard precautions are to be used at all times when coming in contact with blood, bodily fluids, or chemical cleaning agents. Personnel Protective Equipment (PPE) must be worn during each phase of equipment cleaning.

   B. Knowledge of the Occupational Safety and Health Administration (OSHA) rules on occupational exposure to blood-borne pathogens (OSHA Law 29 CRF part 1910).

   C. Knowledge of reprocessing procedures for endoscopes and accessories.

   D. Understanding the mechanisms of disease transmission.

Khashab MA, Robinson TF, Kalloo AN.
The Johns Hopkins Manual for GI Endoscopic Nurses,
Third Edition (pp 15-18).
© 2014 SLACK Incorporated.

E. Maintaining a safe work environment.

F. Safe handling of high-level disinfectants/sterilants.

G. Knowledge of waste management procedures.

2. *Annual updating and training:* It is recommended to have an annual competency program to ensure that personnel are compliant with all protocols. Designated personnel should monitor the adherence to policies and procedures. At our institution, it is a requirement for the cleaning room staff to be certified in Central Sterilization Processing.

3. *Quality assurance:* Infectious disease department is recommended to evaluate the effectiveness of all reprocessing procedures. The cleaning/disinfecting/sterilizing protocols must be evaluated and updated periodically. Endoscope serial numbers must be tracked with patient usage in case of contamination. Patients can be contacted if an issue arises. Most automated endoscope reprocessors (AER) allow entry of patients' medical record numbers to link to endoscope serial numbers. This facilitates easy retrieval of information.

4. *Procedure room management:* The procedure room must be cleaned with Environment Protection Agency (EPA) hospital-grade disinfectant after each procedure and at the end of the day. If the unit accommodates patients with any known or suspected highly transmitted antigens such as *Tuberculosis bacillus,* the unit must be equipped with high-efficiency particulate air (HEPA) filters. It is also recommended to perform these cases at the end of the day to allow adequate time for cleaning of the room and for complete air exchange via filters.

5. *Cleaning room management:* Endoscopes are to be cleaned in an area separate from the procedure rooms. However, pre-cleaning can be performed in the procedure room:

A. Adequate air flow and ventilation per OSHA guidelines for cleaning room air quality

B. Large surfaces to accommodate separate "clean" and "dirty" work areas

C. Adequate lighting

D. Water supply with at least drinking water quality and sufficient pressure for washer filter function

E. Air-drying capability

F. An independent sink for hand washing

G. Eye washing station

H. Hospital-specific spill containment protocol

Cleaning and Disinfecting Endoscopy Equipment

6. *The Food and Drug Administration (FDA):* The FDA recommends a low-suds enzymatic detergent prewash prior to immersion of the endoscope in a high-level disinfectant/sterilization and 70% isopropyl alcohol. All surfaces are to be cleaned with a hospital-grade EPA-approved disinfectant. Disposable equipment is never to be used. All accessories classified according to depth of mucosal penetration must be disinfected/sterilized according to the manufacturer's guidelines:

   A. Sterilization is required for accessories that break the mucous membrane, contact sterile tissue, or contact the vascular system (eg, biopsy forceps and water bottles). Sterile water is to be used in the water bottle because the scope comes in direct contact with the mucosa during the procedure. Water bottles are to be sterilized.

   B. High-level disinfection is needed for instruments that only contact the mucous membrane (eg, endoscopes).

   C. Low-level disinfection is used for equipment that only contacts the skin (eg, pulse oximeters).

7. *Cleaning and disinfecting:*

   A. Pre-cleaning: Pre-cleaning starts in the procedure room. This is important to rid the scope of bioburden. Use a sponge or lint-free gauze soaked with enzymatic cleaner as the first step to decontaminate the scope from blood, mucus, and feces. The insertion tube and control head should also be wiped down. If the endoscope has an elevator port or a water auxiliary port, flush as per manufacturer's recommendations, even if not used. Suction approximately 200 cc of enzymatic cleaner through insertion tube. Then suction approximately 100 cc of clean water followed by suctioning air. The friction of the liquids and air through the channel can dislodge debris and is the first step to decontamination.

   B. Transfer of scope to cleaning room: After pre-cleaning is completed, disconnect the scope from processor and place in a bin or an alternative carrying device. Place a cover over the bin if using bins. The scope is not to be taken to the cleaning room without a carrier. This will prevent any contaminant from dripping on the floor during transportation of the scope.

   C. The decontamination process continues once the endoscope reaches the cleaning room. Leak testing is the first step to perform. It is vital in avoiding a fluid invasion. A leak test is performed by either wet or dry leak testing depending on the manufacturer. The leak tester is to be evaluated for proper functioning before connecting to the scope. Once connected to the scope, the leak tester is turned on and the scope can then be immersed in the water bath. The scope is inspected for leaks anywhere from the head of the scope to the distal end of the insertion tube. The control knobs are to be turned in different directions to stress the bending section a bit for a comprehensive leak exam. This is wet leak testing. Dry leak testing is performed with a pressure gauge and the scope is not immersed in water. If there is a leak, the pressure will decrease. The scope must be sent for repair if there is a positive leak test.

D. All channels are to be brushed thoroughly and the outside of the endoscope cleaned with enzymatic detergent and water. The channels are to be mechanically or manually flushed with enzymatic cleaner and water. Finally, the scope is to be flushed with clean water and then air. Adhere to manufacturer's recommendations for all steps of gross cleaning the endoscope.

E. After the endoscope has properly been decontaminated, place the scope in an AER.

F. When the AER is complete, remove the scope from the reprocessor and flush the endoscopic channels with compressed air.

G. Endoscopes are to be hung vertically with the valves and protective caps off to ensure fluid drainage and drying process.

H. Insufficient data exist for how long an endoscope can be kept in a cabinet unused. AORN and the Association for Professionals in Infection Control and Epidemiology recommend that the maximal storage intervals without reprocessing to be 5 to 7 days, respectively.

Chapter 5

ENDOSCOPY IN PATIENTS WITH SPECIFIC MEDICAL PROBLEMS

MOUEN A. KHASHAB, MD

Antibiotic prophylaxis for gastrointestinal endoscopic procedures are described in Table 5-1. One acceptable antibiotic prophylaxis regime consists of intravenous ampicillin 2 g and gentamicin 1.5 mg/kg (up to 80 mg) 30 minutes prior to the endoscopic procedure, followed by amoxicillin 1.5 g orally 6 hours after the procedure. For penicillin-sensitive patients, vancomycin or clindamycin may be substituted.

Patients undergoing percutaneous gastrostomy tube placement should receive cefazolin 1 g 30 minutes prior to the procedure. If, however, these patients are already on an equivalent antibiotic, no other antibiotic medications are necessary.

DIABETES MELLITUS

Diabetes mellitus is a metabolic abnormality resulting from insufficient production of insulin by the pancreas, leading to elevated blood glucose levels (hyperglycemia). Blood glucose levels greater than 200 mg/dL, polydipsia, polyuria, fatigue, and weight loss characterize the disease. Special considerations during endoscopy are listed next.

PREPROCEDURE

- Uncomplicated, well-controlled patients should be instructed to take half their normal insulin dose on the day of their procedure. Patients taking oral hypoglycemics should be instructed to omit their morning dose on the day of the procedure.

19

Khashab MA, Robinson TF, Kalloo AN.
The Johns Hopkins Manual for GI Endoscopic Nurses,
Third Edition (pp 19-25).
© 2014 SLACK Incorporated.

TABLE 5-1. ANTIBIOTIC PROPHYLAXIS FOR GASTROINTESTINAL ENDOSCOPIC PROCEDURES

MEDICAL CONDITION	PROCEDURE	PROPHYLAXIS
Prosthetic valve	Stricture dilations	Yes
History of endocarditis	Varix sclerosing	
Systemic pulmonary shunt Synthetic vascular graft	ERCP with obstruction Colonoscopy and EGD with/without biopsy/polypectomy Variceal ligation	Physician's discretion
Rheumatic valve dysfunction Mitral valve prolapse with insufficiency	Stricture dilation Varix sclerosing ERCP with obstruction	Physician's discretion
Cardiomyopathy Congenital cardiac anomaly	Colonoscopy and EGD with/without biopsy/polypectomy	No
All other cardiac conditions (status post coronary artery bypass graft surgery, automatic internal defibrillator, pacemaker)	All endoscopic procedures	No

(continued)

- Check the patient's blood glucose with a glucometer on arrival to the unit.
- Notify the physician if the blood glucose level is below 60 or above 200 mg/dL.

TABLE 5-1. ANTIBIOTIC PROPHYLAXIS FOR GASTROINTESTINAL ENDOSCOPIC PROCEDURES (CONTINUED)		
MEDICAL CONDITION	PROCEDURE	PROPHYLAXIS
Obstructed biliary ducts Pancreatic pseudo-cysts	ERCP	Yes
Cirrhosis and ascites Immunocompromised patients	Stricture dilation Varix sclerosing	Physician's discretion
	Biliary obstruction EGD and colonos-copy with/without biopsy/polypec-tomy	No
Orthoprosthesis	Any procedure	No
All patients	PEG placement	Yes
ERCP = endoscopic retrograde cholangiopancreatography; EGD = esopha-gogastroduodenoscopy; PEG = percutaneus endoscopic gastrostomy		

- The physician may order 50% glucose intravenous (IV) prior to the procedure for levels below 60 mg/dL. Normal saline should be the IV solution of choice for levels above 200 mg/dL

INTRAPROCEDURE

- Changes in vital signs and mental status, including combative behavior, may be a result of changes in the blood sugar level, including hypoglycemia.
- Glucagon, which is used to produce hypotonic bowel, may cause elevations in blood glucose.
- The nurse must be aware of the complications of diabetes. These include myocardial infarction, stroke, kidney failure, poor circulation, hypertension, and heart failure.

POSTPROCEDURE

- The physician should instruct the patient regarding the resumption of insulin or oral hypoglycemic medications.

COAGULOPATHY

Coagulopathy is a pathologic condition that affects the ability of the blood to clot. Special considerations during endoscopy are listed below.

PREPROCEDURE

- Verify patient's current prothrombin time (PT), partial thromboplastin time (PTT), platelet level, and international normalized ratio (INR) if biopsy, dilation, or sphincterotomy are contemplated.
- If PT, PTT, platelet level, or INR are not within normal limits, the physician may order fresh frozen plasma (FFP)/platelets.
- Document the patient's baseline vital signs.
- Document the patient's baseline mental status.

INTRAPROCEDURE

- Have equipment for hemostasis (see Chapter 6, "EGD for Hemostasis in Patients With Upper Gastrointestinal Bleeding") readily available for control of bleeding.

POSTPROCEDURE

- Monitor for signs of bleeding (eg, a significant decrease in blood pressure, increased heart rate, change in mental status, and vomiting blood).

HYPERTENSION

Hypertension is a common, often asymptomatic, disorder associated with a consistently elevated blood pressure exceeding 140/90 mm Hg. Special considerations during endoscopy are listed below.

PREPROCEDURE

- Patients should be advised to take antihypertensive medications as prescribed with a sip of water 2 hours prior to the procedure.
- Document the patient's baseline blood pressure and notify the physician if the pressure is abnormally elevated (above 200 systolic and 100 diastolic).

- D5W (dextrose and water) should be the IV solution of choice or D5/.45 NS (dextrose and half normal saline).

INTRAPROCEDURE

- Monitor blood pressure and titrate sedation appropriately.

POSTPROCEDURE

- Notify the physician if the patient's blood pressure is elevated.

CONGESTIVE HEART FAILURE

Congestive heart failure is a condition of impaired cardiac pumping manifested by pulmonary congestion, systemic venous congestion, and peripheral edema. Special considerations during endoscopy are listed below.

PREPROCEDURE

- Patients should be instructed to take cardiac medications as prescribed with a sip of water 2 hours prior to the procedure.
- Monitor and document baseline vital signs, mental status, and peripheral edema.
- Although electrocardiograms are not required on routine ambulatory cases, they may be ordered selectively based on medical history and physical exam.

INTRAPROCEDURE

- Avoid fluid overload by monitoring intravenous infusions.
- Be alert for changes in the electrocardiogram (EKG).
- Use intravenous solution of choice, D5W or D5/.45 NS.

POSTPROCEDURE

- Monitor and document vital signs, mental status, and peripheral edema.

CARDIAC ARRHYTHMIA

A cardiac arrhythmia is any deviation from the normal cardiac electrical pattern. The heart beat may be too fast or too slow and may be regular or irregular. Special considerations during endoscopy are listed next.

PREPROCEDURE

- The patient should be instructed to take cardiac medications as prescribed with a sip of water 2 hours prior to the procedure.
- Although EKGs are not required on routine ambulatory cases, they may be ordered selectively based on medical history and physical exam.
- If the patient has an automatic internal defibrillator (AID) it should be turned off for the procedure when using electrocautery if working above the diaphragm. If working below the diaphragm, the AID may be left on. However, always follow the policies and procedures of your individual institutions.

INTRAPROCEDURE

- Monitor the EKG for any changes from baseline.
- Have emergency equipment readily accessible.

POSTPROCEDURE

- If the patient has EKG changes during the procedure, EKG monitoring should be continued along with monitoring of other vital signs.
- Reinstate the internal defibrillator if appropriate.

PULMONARY INSUFFICIENCY

Pulmonary insufficiency is a prolonged or persistent condition of respiratory dysfunction resulting in insufficient oxygenation or carbon dioxide elimination to meet the demands of the body. Special considerations during endoscopy are listed below.

PREPROCEDURE

- Assess baseline respiratory status.
- Determine if patient is a "CO_2 retainer."
- If the patient is wheezing, a metaproterenol nebulizer may be required before the procedure.

INTRAPROCEDURE

- Oxygen delivery should be maintained at 2 L except for in CO_2 retainers, who may require less or no supplemental oxygen.
- Monitor the patient for coughing, wheezing, dyspnea, and shortness of breath.

- If the patient is wheezing, a metaproterenol nebulizer may be required before the procedure.
- Make sure the patient is positioned properly to enhance maximum lung capacity:
  ▷ Elevate the patient's head and chest slightly (approximately 30 degrees)
  ▷ Secure proper body alignment so the torso is straight

POSTPROCEDURE

- Monitor respiratory status.
- If the patient is wheezing, a metaproterenol nebulizer may be required.
- If required, oxygen may be administered.

RENAL INSUFFICIENCY

Renal insufficiency is a loss of kidney function and diminishes the ability to excrete wastes, concentrate urine, and conserve electrolytes. Special considerations during endoscopy are listed below.

PREPROCEDURE

- Dialysis patients should be scheduled for endoscopic procedures just before regular dialysis treatment.
- If the patient has a dialysis shunt or subclavian central line, avoid using that arm for blood pressure, intravenous fluids, or administration of medications.

INTRAPROCEDURE

- Monitor intravenous fluids carefully to prevent fluid overload.
- Monitor the amount of sedation the patient is receiving since he or she may have difficulty excreting the medication.

POSTPROCEDURE

- Monitor urine output (have the patient void before discharge from the unit).
- Be aware of the complications of renal insufficiency (eg, hypertension, poor circulation, diabetes mellitus, or a change in mental status).

Chapter 6

Diagnostic and Therapeutic Endoscopic Procedures

Diagnostic Esophagogastroduodenoscopy

Mouen A. Khashab, MD

Esophagogastroduodenoscopy (EGD) refers to the endoscopic examination of the esophagus, stomach, and the first and second portions of the small intestine for the purpose of diagnosis and treatment of disorders of the upper gastrointestinal (GI) tract.

Equipment (Figure 6-1)

- Upper endoscope
- Light source
- Sterile water bottle and sterile water
- Biopsy forceps (Figure 6-2)
- Bite block (Figure 6-3)
- Topical anesthetic
- Suction equipment (Figure 6-4)

Additional Equipment That May Be Needed

- Bottles of formalin for biopsy specimens
- Labels with patient's name and pathology requisitions
- Cytology brushes (Figure 6-5)

Khashab MA, Robinson TF, Kalloo AN.
*The Johns Hopkins Manual for GI Endoscopic Nurses,
Third Edition* (pp 27-220).
© 2014 SLACK Incorporated.

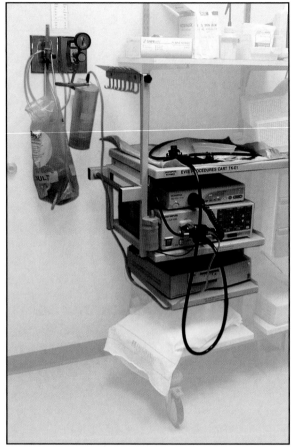

Figure 6-1. Endoscopy set-up.

- Viral and fungal culture tubes
- Mucus trap (Figure 6-6)

Nursing Implications

Preprocedure

- The patient should have nothing by mouth (NPO) for 8 hours prior to the procedure.
- Document baseline blood pressure, pulse, respirations, oxygen saturation, level of consciousness, and pain level.

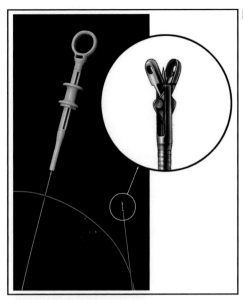

Figure 6-2. Biopsy forceps.

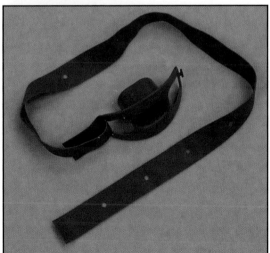

Figure 6-3. Bite block.

Figure 6-4. Suction apparatus.

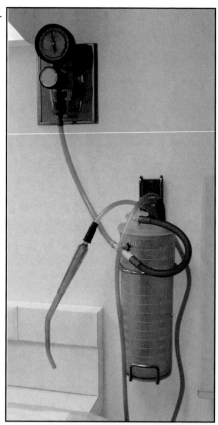

- Document drug allergies and daily medications, including dose and frequency.
- Discontinue aspirin and nonsteroidal anti-inflammatory drugs (NSAIDs) for 1 week prior to the procedure.
- Start IV of D5/.45 NS (normal saline) or .9 normal saline.
- The physician should obtain an informed consent from the patient or responsible adult.
- Obtain medical history from the patient or responsible adult and confirm the completion of a physical exam by the physician.
- Review the discharge instructions with the patient or responsible adult before sedation is administered.
- Ensure that a responsible adult is available to accompany the patient home.

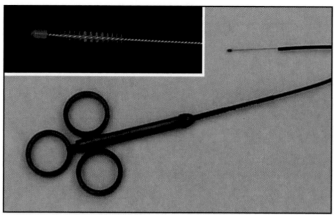

Figure 6-5. Cytology brush.

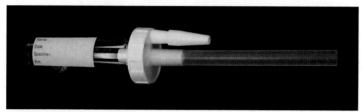

Figure 6-6. Mucus trap.

INTRAPROCEDURE

- Patient positioning (Figure 6-7):
  - ▷ Use left lateral position to facilitate drainage of pharyngeal secretions.
  - ▷ Knees should be bent toward the chest for comfort and stabilization of the patient.
  - ▷ The patient's head may be flexed in a forward position to ease the introduction of the endoscope.
- Patient monitoring:
  - ▷ Document electrocardiogram (EKG), blood pressure, respiratory rate, and pulse oximetry every 2 minutes during administration of sedation.
  - ▷ Document EKG, blood pressure, respiratory rate, and pulse oximetry every 15 minutes during the procedure or more often if the patient's condition warrants.
  - ▷ Pain level must be monitored during the procedure.

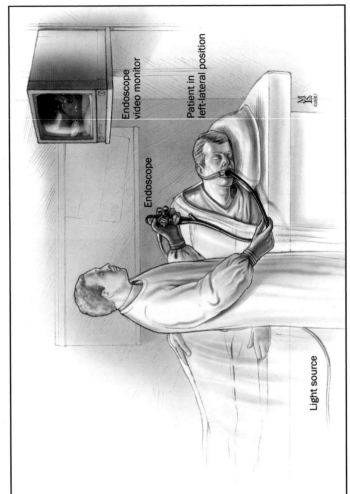

Figure 6-7. Endoscopy set-up.

- ▷ Emergency equipment, including suction, oxygen, and crash cart, must be readily available.
- Topical anesthetic:
  - ▷ Viscous lidocaine swish and swallow or 4% lidocaine spray may be used.
- Additional comfort measures:
  - ▷ Place a pillow behind the patient's back for extra support while on his or her side.
  - ▷ Soothing, calming words of encouragement along with light back massage may improve the patient's comfort.

POSTPROCEDURE

- Keep the patient on the left side until fully awake and able to control secretions.
- Monitor vital signs, blood pressure, pulse, oxygen saturation, level of consciousness, and pain level until they have returned to baseline.
- The patient may be discharged home, accompanied by an adult with discharge instructions (see Appendix 2).
- The physician should be notified if the patient experiences vomiting, abdominal pain, distension, or fever.

Chapter 6

EGD WITH DILATION FOR
ESOPHAGEAL STRICTURES
David W. Victor III, MD

Dilation therapy is performed in the upper GI tract for the following conditions: achalasia, surgically or chemically induced esophageal and pyloric strictures, and webs or rings. The instruments used to dilate strictures include balloons (through-the-scope [TTS] and over-the-guidewire), mercury bougienage (Maloney) dilators, botulinum toxin injection, and hollow polyvinyl (Savary) dilators (Figure 6-8).

The type of instrument used is dependent upon the severity of the stricture. Mild to moderately tight strictures can be dilated with a TTS balloon. Fluoroscopy is seldom required, and the risk of perforation is low in cases of benign strictures. Maloney dilators may also be used for this type of stricture. The physician proceeds by beginning with a dilator that can be passed through the stricture with mild resistance and continues to increase the dilator size up to three sizes in succession ("rule of threes"). The physician may continue to increase the dilator size provided that the resistance is mild to moderate.

Achalasia and Savary dilators, both over-the-guidewire, are typically used with fluoroscopy. The achalasia dilator is used only for patients with achalasia (a motility disorder of the esophagus resulting in failure of the lower esophageal sphincter [LES] to relax). The balloon dilators are available in a variety of sizes: 30, 35, 40, and 45 mm. The Savary dilator is used for tight strictures that prohibit passage of a Maloney dilator. At times strictures are injected with steroids after physical dilation to increase the efficacy of dilation.

Botulinum toxin is a potent neuromuscular blocker. It is injected in the upper GI tract to relax smooth muscle and allows for muscular strictures to dilate.

The endoscope is initially passed to assess the tightness of the stricture. When using the Maloney dilator, the endoscope is withdrawn and the dilator blindly passed, guided by the endoscopist's finger placed into the patient's pharynx. TTS dilators are passed through the biopsy channel of the endoscope and then inflated (Figure 6-9). Both Savary and achalasia dilators are passed over a guidewire after the endoscope is withdrawn. Achalasia dilators demonstrate a "waist" on fluoroscopy that disappears upon inflation of the balloon (Figure 6-10). The radiopaque-marked Savary dilators can be followed through the stricture with the use of fluoroscopy.

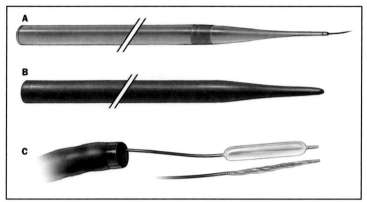

Figure 6-8. Dilators used for esophageal dilation: (A) Savary dilator, (B) Maloney dilator, and (C) "through-the-scope" dilator.

EQUIPMENT FOR SAVARY DILATION

- Same as for a diagnostic EGD.
- A pediatric endoscope may be used depending upon the tightness of the stricture.
- A large-bore mouth piece may be needed to accommodate a 20-mm dilator.
- Savary dilators and guidewire (Savary guidewire or any .038-inch diameter guidewire per physician's preference) (Figures 6-11 and 6-12).
- Fluoroscopy
- Water-soluble lubricant

EQUIPMENT FOR THROUGH-THE-SCOPE DILATION

- Same as for a diagnostic EGD.
- A pediatric endoscope may be used depending upon the tightness of the stricture.
- TTS balloons (10 to 20 mm)
- Dilating gun and adapter with pressure gauge and syringe (Figure 6-13)
- Water for insufflation of balloon
- Lubricant if needed

EQUIPMENT FOR MALONEY DILATION

- Same as for a diagnostic EGD.

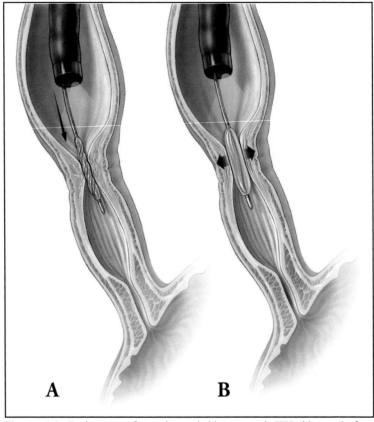

Figure 6-9. Technique of esophageal dilation with TTS dilators before (A) and after (B) stricture dilation.

- A pediatric endoscope may be used depending upon the tightness of the stricture.
- Maloney dilators (36 to 60 mm, increasing in 4-mm increments)
- Water or water-soluble lubricant

EQUIPMENT FOR STEROID OR BOTULINUM TOXIN INJECTION DILATION

- Same as for diagnostic EGD.
- Steroid or botulinum toxic should be ordered from pharmacy/Pyxis (CareFusion) prior to procedure

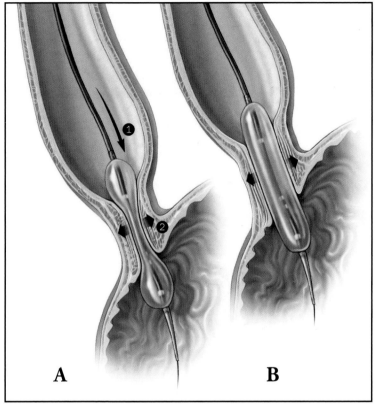

Figure 6-10. Technique of pneumatic dilation before (A) and after (B) dilation.

- Further information available in the section "Botulinum Toxin Injection in the Upper Gastrointestinal Tract" on p. 206
- Sclerotherapy needle
- Injection is done in standard fashion and dosage should be adjusted as per the physician

EQUIPMENT FOR ACHALASIA DILATION

- Same as for a diagnostic EGD.
- A pediatric endoscope may be used depending upon the tightness of the stricture.
- Fluoroscopy
- Radiopaque .038-inch diameter guidewire

Figure 6-11. Standard esophageal guidewire.

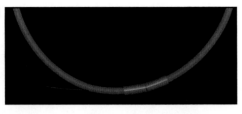

Figure 6-12. Savary guidewire.

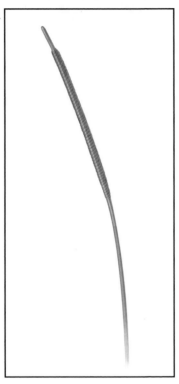

- Over-the-guidewire achalasia balloon dilators (30, 35, 40, and 45 mm)
- Radiopaque half-strength contrast (50 cc distilled water plus 50 cc ionic contrast)
- Water and water-soluble lubricant for lubrication of dilator

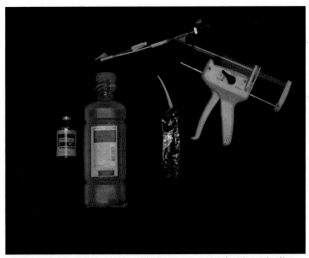

Figure 6-13. Pneumatic dilator gun attached to balloon with agents for balloon sufflation.

NURSING IMPLICATIONS

PREPROCEDURE

- Same as for a diagnostic EGD.
- Anticoagulant therapy may be adjusted or discontinued on the advice of the physician.
- Prophylactic antibiotics (if indicated).
- Patients undergoing achalasia dilation should have clear liquids for 24 to 36 hours prior to the procedure since retained food may be present in the esophagus even after a 12-hour fast.

INTRAPROCEDURE

- Same as for a diagnostic EGD.
- The patient should be positioned on the fluoroscopy table for Savary or achalasia dilations. Fluoroscopy may be necessary for guidewire placement.
- Savary dilation: The physician may require assistance with the guidewire. The nurse should keep the end of the guidewire coiled and taut while the dilator is passed. The guidewire should not be allowed to slide forward or backward during insertion or removal by paying attention to the guidewire markings.

- TTS dilation: The nurse will be asked to inflate the balloon to the appropriate pressure. Inflation duration is dependent on the discretion of the physician.
- Maloney dilation: The nurse should support the distal end of the dilator during insertion by the physician.
- Achalasia dilation: Patient comfort and compliance are aided by bolus sedation immediately before balloon inflation (because of increased pain during dilation).
- Patient monitoring: Same as for a diagnostic EGD.
- Topical anesthetic: Same as for a diagnostic EGD.
- Additional comfort measures: Same as for a diagnostic EGD.
- Some bleeding and increased pharyngeal fluid may be expected during dilation. Frequent suctioning is imperative to prevent aspiration.

POSTPROCEDURE

- Same as for a diagnostic EGD.
- Patients should be monitored for symptoms and signs of perforation (chest pain, difficulty breathing or swallowing, or presence of subcutaneous air) following dilation. The risk of perforation is higher in achalasia dilation.
- The patient should be able to take fluid by mouth without difficulty or pain prior to discharge.
- Radiologic studies may be required after dilation if the patient exhibits symptoms or signs of perforation

EGD FOR HEMOSTASIS IN PATIENTS WITH UPPER GASTROINTESTINAL BLEEDING

UGI

Eduardo Gonzalez-Velez, MD

EGD may be performed to control upper GI bleeding. The most common causes of acute upper GI bleeding include gastric and duodenal ulcers, esophageal varices, gastritis, duodenitis, Mallory-Weiss tears, gastric antral vascular ectasia (GAVE), and arteriovenous malformations (AVMs).

EQUIPMENT

- Large or double-channel upper endoscope (to facilitate the aspiration of blood) (Figure 6-14)
- Bipolar cautery probe with electrosurgical cautery unit (Figure 6-15)
- Argon plasma coagulator (APC) (Figure 6-16)
- Sclerotherapy needle with injectable agents (such as saline, epinephrine, or sodium morrhuate or other sclerosing agents) (Figure 6-17)
- Clipping device (Endoclips vary in diameter when open, permitting the closing of various sized defects. Some have the ability to rotate. The over-the-scope clipping [OTSC] system can be used to achieve hemostasis for large ulcers and to close perforations. [Figure 6-18])
- Variceal band ligator (Figure 6-19)
- Suction equipment

NURSING IMPLICATIONS

PREPROCEDURE

- Same as for a diagnostic EGD.
- Gastric lavage may be ordered to clear the stomach of blood and food in emergent situations.
- IV infusion of erythromycin (prokinetic) 250 mg, 30 min. before endoscopy could be ordered to clear stomach contents and improve visualization during endoscopy.
- Patients presenting with suspected upper GI bleeding due to peptic ulcer disease are treated with IV proton pump inhibitor (80-mg bolus followed by 8 mg/hr.). This results in a decrease of

UGI

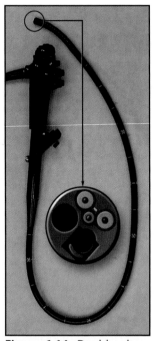

Figure 6-14. Double channel (therapeutic) endoscope.

the proportion of patients with high risk lesions that will require endoscopic intervention.

- Patients with cirrhosis and upper GI bleeding are prescribed fluoroquinolone or ceftriaxone, depending on local antibiotic pattern of resistance, for prevention of bacterial infections due to translocation. Pharmacological therapy with somatostatin analogue (octreotide) is initiated as soon as variceal hemorrhage is suspected and continued for 3 to 5 days after endoscopic therapy.

INTRAPROCEDURE

- Same as for a diagnostic EGD.
- Patient positioning: Same as for a diagnostic EGD.
- Patient monitoring: Same as for a diagnostic EGD.
- Topical anesthetic: Same as for a diagnostic EGD.
- Additional comfort measures: Same as for a diagnostic EGD.

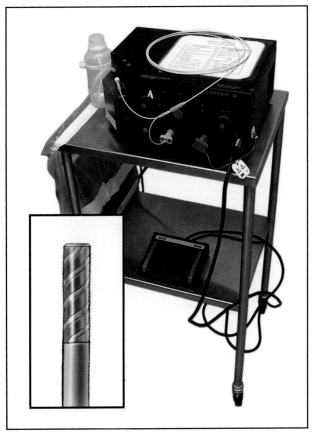

Figure 6-15. Electrosurgical unit with cautery probe.

- Endoscopic therapy of bleeding due to peptic ulcer disease depends on the characteristic of the lesion found. Ulcers with high risk stigmata for rebleeding (such as active bleeding, oozing of blood, visible vessel, and adherent clots) should be treated endoscopically. Combination therapy is advised and the use of epinephrine injection as the only treatment modality for peptic ulcer disease with high risk features is not recommended.
- Biopsies of the gastric mucosa can be performed to assess for the presence of *Helicobacter pylori* in patients with peptic ulcer disease.

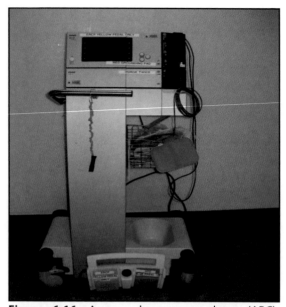

Figure 6-16. Argon plasma coagulator (APC). Components are argon compatible, high frequency monopolar electrosurgical generator, APC unit, Argon gas source, foot activation switch, and delivery catheters. The electrical current and argon gas are synchronized with the use of the foot switch. Anatomical location of the lesions determines the power setting. Gastric, duodenal, and left colonic lesions were treated at 60 W, whereas small intestine, right colon, and cecum were treated with 40 W, given the thin bowel wall in the latter locations. Argon gas flow ranged from 2 to 2.5 L/min. If APC is going to be applied to lesions in the colon, the patient must have a full colonoscopy preparation in order to reduce the risk of explosion secondary to ignition of retained colonic methane or hydrogen. The settings on the APC should be visualized and verbally confirmed with the physician. The patient's abdomen has to be frequently examined to assess for distension. During the procedure the probe is cleansed from debris and inspected for damage. Treating GAVE, arteriovenous malformation (AVM), and radiation proctitis are some of the indications for the APC.

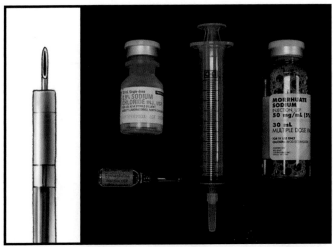

Figure 6-17. Sclerotherapy needle with agents used for injection.

POSTPROCEDURE

- Same as for a diagnostic EGD.
- After endoscopic therapy for high risk of re-bleeding peptic ulcer disease, proton pump inhibitor infusion is continued at 8 mg/hour for 72 hours.
- Patients who have undergone esophageal variceal band ligation should be placed on nonselective beta blockers (propanolol or nadolol), if possible, for prophylaxis against recurrent esophageal variceal hemorrhage.

UGI

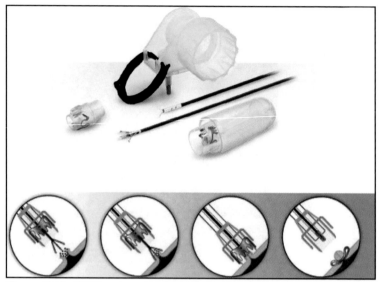

Figure 6-18. OTSC system: hemostasis for large ulcers or perforations.

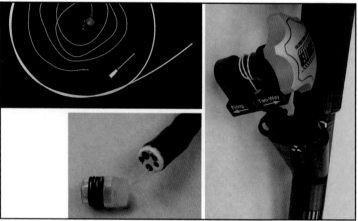

Figure 6-19. Typical band ligation equipment and set-up.

EGD FOR REMOVAL OF
FOREIGN OBJECTS AND FOOD BOLUS

Eduardo Gonzalez-Velez, MD

UGI

Most foreign body ingestions are accidental, with most cases involving children 6 months to 6 years of age. Adults with psychiatric disorders, alcohol intoxication, and prisoners are frequently involved in nonfood object ingestion. A myriad of foreign body ingestions have been described in the literature, ranging from coins, batteries, forks, toothbrushes, and paper clips to name a few. Complications from foreign body ingestion are aspiration, perforation, mediastinitis, bleeding, and fistula formation.

Guidelines for the endoscopic removal of these objects have been published. Recommendations on the appropriate management depend on the size, shape, number of objects, location in the GI track, and time of ingestion. History will help disclose the type of object, time since ingestion, and symptoms. Patient can present with choking, refusal to eat, drooling, and respiratory distress. Odynophagia or sore throat could be experienced but the patient could also present completely asymptomatic.

Altered vital signs could indicate serious complications such as perforation by the foreign body. During the initial evaluation the physician and nurse should also be attentive for signs of proximal esophageal perforation, which can lead to neck swelling, tenderness, and crepitus. Signs and symptoms associated with peritonitis should also be noticed immediately on evaluation since management would be surgical if present before endoscopy is performed.

Airway assessment is crucial to determine if general anesthesia requiring endotracheal entubation to protect airway from aspiration is needed. History, physical exam, and imaging studies ordered could also dictate the use of general anesthesia. Most of the pediatric population, uncooperative patients, patients with multiple or complex foreign bodies, and food boluses in whom the removal would be prolonged are candidates for general anesthesia.

Diagnostic imaging in the form of x-ray plain films anterior and lateral of the neck, thorax and abdomen aid in determining the size, shape, number of objects, and location. Signs of perforation can also be documented on x-rays such as free air and subcuteanous emphysema. Barium or contrast studies should be avoided due to the risk of aspiration, and oral contrast could subsequently hamper endoscopic visualization of the foreign body.

Upper endoscopy timing for removal is dependent on these factors. Refer to Table 6-1.

Conservative management can be ordered by a physician depending on the shape, size, and location of the foreign body in the GI tract. Asymptomatic patients who ingested a small blunt object are instructed to continue regular diet and observe their stools for evidence of passage. In the absence of symptoms, weekly radiographs are sufficient to monitor small blunt object as it can take 4 weeks for them to pass. Sharp pointed objects that have passed to the small bowel without complications are followed by serial x-rays. Patients are placed on a high-fiber diet, but laxatives should be avoided. Patients are instructed to screen stools, but if on imaging, the object fails to progress in 3 to 4 days, surgery is entertained.

In the Western world, the most common foreign body in the esophagus of adults is food bolus impaction. Pharmacotherapy in this population can play a role with the use of glucagon at the discretion of the physician. Glucagon causes relaxation of the LES, which could lead to the passage of the food bolus into the stomach. The standard dose is 1 to 2 mg intravenously and may be repeated in 5 to 10 min. Slow administration could help avoid hyperglycemia, which is one of the side effects. Other common side effects are nausea and vomiting. This medication is contraindicated in patients with insulinoma, pheochromocytoma, Zollinger Ellison syndrome, and known hypersensitivity to glucagon. Enzyme preparation and gas-forming agent to aid with passage of food impactions are no longer recommended due to the risk of perforation.

Patients who present with food bolus impaction in the esophagus usually have an underlying pathology that predisposes the individual to this event. Schatzki ring or peptic stricture are some pathologies that could be treated after the food bolus impaction is removed, if underlying mucosa reveals no signs of inflammation. Part of the equipment to have available in the endoscopy unit is that used for dilation. A frequent cause of food impaction in young adults is eosinophilic esophagitis for which biopsy forceps for mid and distal sampling of the esophagus would be taken.

Education after discharge for the patient with food impaction includes adequate chewing technique and ingesting small portions of food. Food impaction in the edentulous would warrant evaluation with dentistry for dentures.

TABLE 6-1. TIMING OF ENDOSCOPY FOR INGESTED FOREIGN BODIES

EMERGENT ENDOSCOPY

- Patients with esophageal obstruction (ie, unable to manage secretions)
- Disk batteries in the esophagus
- Sharp-pointed objects in the esophagus

URGENT ENDOSCOPY

- Esophageal foreign objects that are not sharp
- Esophageal food impaction in patients without complete obstruction
- Sharp pointed objects in the stomach or duodenum
- Objects >5 cm in length or above the proximal duodenum
- Magnets within endoscopic reach

NON-URGENT ENDOSCOPY

- Coins in the esophagus may be observed for 12 to 24 hours before endoscopic removal in an asymptomatic patient
- Objects in the stomach with diameter >2.5 cm
- Disk batteries and cylindrical batteries that are in the stomach of patients without signs of GI injury may be observed for as long as 48 hours. Batteries remaining in the stomach longer than 48 hours should be removed.

EQUIPMENT

- Double-channel upper endoscope (to facilitate the aspiration of blood) (see Figure 6-14). Use a 5.9- to 6-mm upper endoscope, colonoscope, double balloon enteroscope)
- Overtube (esophageal length, gastric length [Figure 6-20])
- Bell shape latex hood (Figure 6-21)
- Foreign body forceps (Grasping forceps: V shape [Figure 6-22], rat tooth [Figure 6-23], alligator jaw [Figure 6-24], pentapod [Figure 6-25])

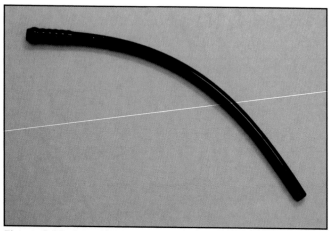

Figure 6-20. Overtube.

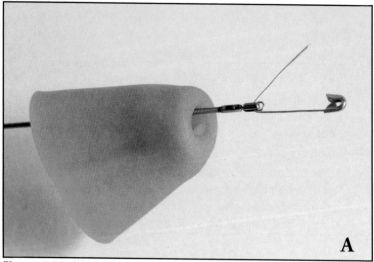

Figure 6-21. (A) Bell shape latex hood offers protection against sharp objects as hood is inverted to cover the sharp object when retrieving the object from the stomach into the esophagus.

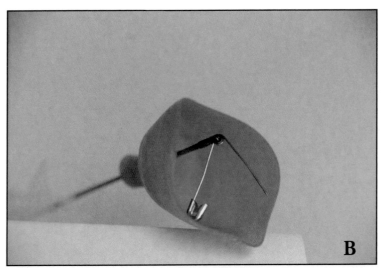

B

Figure 6-21. (B) Bell shape latex hood offers protection against sharp objects as hood is inverted to cover the sharp object when retrieving the object from the stomach into the esophagus.

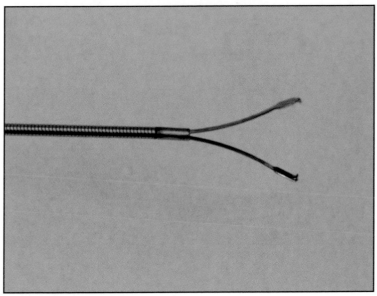

Figure 6-22. Grasping forcep: V shape.

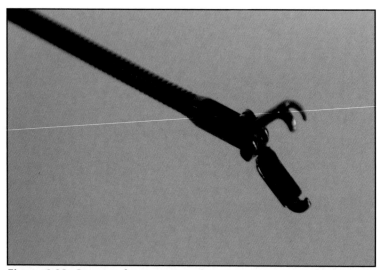

Figure 6-23. Grasping forcep: rat tooth.

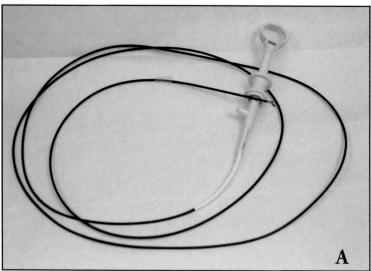

Figure 6-24. (A) Grasping forcep: alligator jaw.

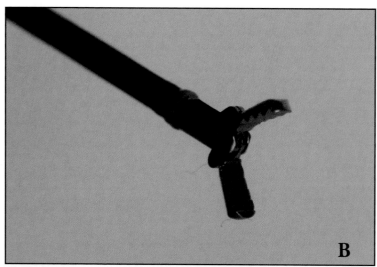

B

Figure 6-24. (B) Grasping forcep: alligator jaw close-up.

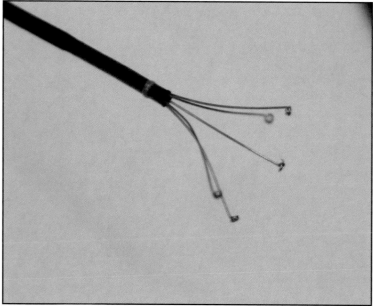

Figure 6-25. Grasping forcep: pentapod.

- Polypectomy snare
- Roth retrieval net
- Friction fit adaptor (EMR, variceal band ligator)
- Dormia basket
- Grasping forceps (Magil, Kelly)
- Suction equipment

NURSING IMPLICATIONS

PREPROCEDURE

- Same as for a diagnostic EGD.

INTRAPROCEDURE

- Same as for a diagnostic EGD.
- Patient positioning: Same as for a diagnostic EGD.
- Patient monitoring: Same as for a diagnostic EGD.
- Topical anesthetic: Same as for a diagnostic EGD.
- Additional comfort measures: Same as for a diagnostic EGD.

POSTPROCEDURE

- Same as for a diagnostic EGD.

EGD With Polypectomy
Mouen A. Khashab, MD

Gastric polyps in the stomach should be removed since the size, distribution, or number of polyps does not reliably differentiate adenomatous from non-neoplastic polyps. Removal may be performed endoscopically using standard hot biopsy forceps or cautery snare techniques.

EQUIPMENT

- Same as for a diagnostic EGD
- Biopsy forceps
- Standard polypectomy snare; looping and clipping devices are also available to assist in hemostasis (Figure 6-26)
- Bipolar/monopolar electrosurgical cautery unit with grounding pad and cautery probe (Figure 6-27)
- Tripod grasping forceps or Roth basket (United States Endoscopy Group Inc) for polyp retrieval (Figures 6-28 and 6-29)
- Mucus trap (to capture smaller polyps instead of using the tripod grasping forceps)
- Epinephrine 1:1000 (in a 10-cc syringe mixed with 9 cc of saline for a dilution of 1:10,000) and sclerotherapy needle (the physician may wish to inject the base of the polyp before removal to reduce the risk of bleeding)

NURSING IMPLICATIONS

PREPROCEDURE

- Same as for a diagnostic EGD.
- Give prophylactic antibiotics (if indicated).
- Anticoagulant therapy may be adjusted or discontinued on the advice of the physician.

INTRAPROCEDURE

- Patient positioning: Same as for a diagnostic EGD.
- Patient monitoring: Same as for a diagnostic EGD.
- Topical anesthetic: Same as for a diagnostic EGD.
- Additional comfort measures: Same as for a diagnostic EGD.

UGI

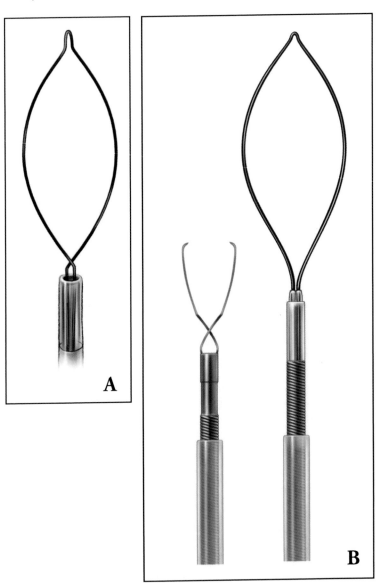

Figure 6-26. (A) Polypectomy snare. (B) Clipping and snare device.

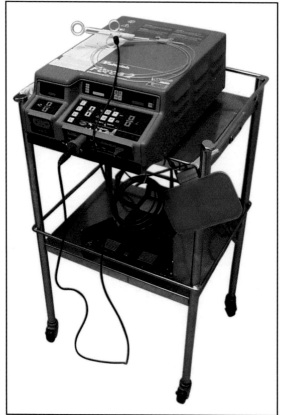

Figure 6-27. Electrosurgical cautery unit with grounding pad and snare.

POSTPROCEDURE

- Same as for a diagnostic EGD.
- The patient should be advised to adhere to a soft diet for 24 hours after polyp removal to prevent mechanical abrasion to the excised area.
- The patient should be instructed to avoid any medications that may increase the risk of bleeding (eg, aspirin) for 1 week after the procedure on the direction of the physician.

UGI

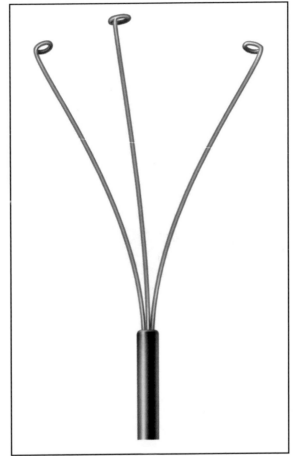

Figure 6-28. Tripod grasping forceps.

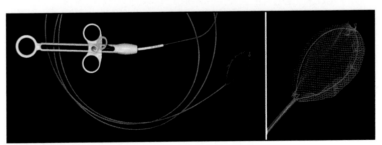

Figure 6-29. Roth basket.

EGD With Narrow Band Imaging
Eun Ji Shin, MD

Narrow band imaging (NBI) is a lighting system based on narrowing the bandwidth of transmitted light using optical filters. This allows fewer wavelengths of light within the RGB (red, green, blue) spectrum to pass through the optical fibers of the endoscope. Blue light, a shorter wavelength, penetrates only the superficial layers, improving imaging resolution. This technology is useful in the early detection of dysplasia of Barrett's esophagus especially if used in combination with topical application of acetic acid, a mucolytic.

EQUIPMENT

- Same as for diagnostic EGD except for the narrow band imaging endoscope (Olympus GIFQ240Z; Olympus America) (Figure 6-30)
- Spray catheter
- 20-cc syringe
- 10 cc normal saline
- 10 cc 5% acetic acid

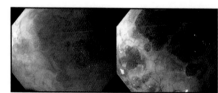

Figure 6-30. Narrow band imaging.

Chapter 6

Nursing Implications

PREPROCEDURE

- Same as for diagnostic EGD.

INTRAPROCEDURE

- Same as for diagnostic EGD.
- Acetic acid preparation:
  - ▷ Put 10 cc 5% acetic acid mixed with 10 cc normal saline in a 20-cc syringe.
  - ▷ Insert spray catheter through the biopsy channel of the endoscope and spray the affected area as directed by the physician.

POSTPROCEDURE

- Same as for diagnostic EGD.

CONFOCAL LASER ENDOMICROSCOPY

Marcia Irene Canto, MD, MHS

Confocal laser endomicroscopy (CLE) is an endoscopic procedure that enables the surface of the intestinal or gastric mucosa to be examined microscopically in vivo during the endoscopy. CLE enables visualization of the cellular, vascular, and connective structures with maximum magnifying power of 1000x. It also enables quantitative measurements of surface mucosa in both lateral and vertical dimensions. Using point scanning laser analysis, the physician is able to have a real-time diagnosis of different GI conditions such as Barrett's esophagus, esophageal and gastric cancer, *Helicobacter pylori* gastritis, colon cancer and ulcerative colitis, collagenous and microscopic colitis, and graft-versus-host disease.

There are two types of CLE. One using a probe passed through the channel of the endoscope (pCLE) and another using a conventional endoscope with built-in small confocal microscope (Figure 6-31) at the distal tip.

EQUIPMENT

- Set up confocal endoscope and processors according to manufacturer's instructions (Pentax EC-3870CIK; Pentax Medical Company)
- Fluorescein 5 mg, contrast agent, frequently used in ophthalmology, is injected intravenously during the endoscopy procedure to enable fluorescence CLE
- 10-cc syringe

NURSING IMPLICATIONS

PREPROCEDURE

- Same as for diagnostic EGD.
- Assess patient for allergies.
- Instruct patient on side effects of fluorescein; yellow skin and eyes for several hours after the procedure, contact lenses should not be worn until the following day, and urine may be bright orange or yellow in color for 12 to 15 hours after the injection of the fluorescein.

Figure 6-31. Confocal scope.

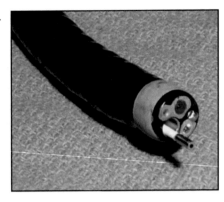

INTRAPROCEDURE

- Same as for diagnostic EGD.
- Prepare fluorescein 5 mg to be given slowly via IV push.
- Monitor patient for adverse side effects such as:
  - ▷ Common:
    - › Cardiovascular: Hypotension, syncope
    - › GI: Drug-induced GI disturbance such as nausea, altered taste sense, and vomiting
    - › Immunologic: Generalized pruritus, hives
    - › Neurologic: Headache
    - › Respiratory: Bronchospasm
  - ▷ Serious:
    - › Cardiovascular: Arterial ischemia, cardiac arrest, shock (severe)
    - › Dermatologic: Injection site; thrombophlebitis
  - ▷ Immunologic:
    - › Anaphylaxis
  - ▷ Neurologic:
    - › Seizure

POSTPROCEDURE

- Same as for diagnostic EGD.
- Assess possible allergic reaction.

Barrett's Ablation With RFA

Eun Ji Shin, MD

Barrett's esophagus is when abnormal intestinal-type epithelium replaces the normal squamous epithelium that lines the esophagus, typically as a consequence of chronic gastroesophageal reflux disease (GERD). It is a predisposing condition to the development of esophageal adenocarcinoma.

Radiofrequency ablation (RFA) is an endoscopic technique that delivers a precise amount of radiofrequency energy to cause coagulation injury to result in a full-thickness mucosal ablation of the Barrett's epithelium. There are two types of RFA devices: the circumferential balloon-based catheter (HALO[360]) and the focal devices (HALO[90] and HALO[60]).

Equipment for Circumferential RFA

- Same as for a diagnostic EGD
- 60-cc syringe with 1% N-Acetylcysteine
- 0.035" extra stiff guidewire
- Soft distal attachment cap for endoscope
- HALO[360] sizing balloon
- HALO[360] ablation catheters in different sizes
- HALO[FLEX] generator

Nursing Implications

Preprocedure

- Same as for diagnostic EGD, except for preparation of RFA unit, which should be set up according to the manufacturer's instructions.

Intraprocedure

- Patient positioning: Same as for a diagnostic EGD.
- Patient monitoring: Same as for a diagnostic EGD.
- Additional comfort measures: Same as for a diagnostic EGD.
- Soft distal attachment cap needs to be affixed to the end of the EGD for cleaning in between the two RFA cycles.

POSTPROCEDURE

- Same as for a diagnostic EGD.
- Diet should consist of liquids for the first 24 hours, progressing to solid foods as tolerated.
- Medications
  ▷ High dose BID proton-pump inhibitor (PPI)
  ▷ Carafate 1 g PO Q6hr PRN (1 hour before meals and at bedtime)
  ▷ Post ablation pain: analgesics
- If necessary, make appointment for subsequent therapy.

EQUIPMENT FOR FOCAL RFA

- Same as for a diagnostic EGD
- 60-cc syringe with 1% N-Acetylcysteine
- HALO^{90} ablation catheter
- HALO^{FLEX} generator

NURSING IMPLICATIONS

PREPROCEDURE

- Same as for diagnostic EGD, except for preparation of RFA unit which should be set up according to the manufacturers' instructions.

INTRAPROCEDURE

- Patient positioning: Same as for a diagnostic EGD.
- Patient monitoring: Same as for a diagnostic EGD.
- Additional comfort measures: Same as for a diagnostic EGD.

POSTPROCEDURE

- Same as for a diagnostic EGD.
- Diet should consist of liquids for the first 24 hours, progressing to solid foods as tolerated.
- Medications
  ▷ High dose BID PPI
  ▷ Carafate 1 g PO Q6hr PRN (1 hour before meals and at bedtime)
  ▷ Postablation pain: analgesics
- If necessary, make appointment for subsequent therapy.

EGD WITH CRYOTHERAPY
Marcia Irene Canto, MD, MHS

Also called cryoablation, cryotherapy is the application of extreme cold to the GI mucosa with either a high pressure device using nitrous oxide gas or a low pressure device using liquid nitrogen at ambient pressure. Cryoablation is performed to destroy the dysplasia and superficial early carcinoma in Barrett's esophagus, provide hemostasis of GI bleeding (ie, watermelon stomach), and palliation of esophageal and gastric neoplasms. The freezing of the tissue allows destruction of the tissue while preserving the underlying collagen tissue to provide a scaffold for healthy tissue to grow. The injury of cryotherapy is both immediate and delayed, unlike thermal injury from energy involving heat (coagulation) such as radiofrequency ablation, multipolar coagulation, or argon plasma coagulation.

There are 2 types of cryotherapy. One type involves administration of liquid nitrogen (which expands rapidly to nitrogen gas) (truFreeze, CSA Medical, Inc) and the other involves delivery of compressed carbon dioxide gas (Polar Wand, GI Supply). The delivery systems of both types of cryotherapy are flexible, allowing application of the cryogen even in retroflex position.

LIQUID NITROGEN CRYOTHERAPY

The liquid nitrogen is delivered through a specially designed heated catheter that lowers the catheter temperature to extremely cold temperatures (-196° C) while liquid nitrogen is sprayed onto the surface of the GI mucosa (CSA Medical, Inc). The catheter is passed through the biopsy channel of the endoscope. A large bore 16 French nasogastric tube with multiple side holes is also placed into the esophagus and stomach to allow suctioning of excess gas resulting from expansion of the liquid nitrogen.

CARBON DIOXIDE CRYOTHERAPY

A catheter with a 0.035-inch opening at the tip (forward spraying) is passed through the biopsy channel of a standard endoscope. The catheter can deliver pressure of 450 to 750 psi. Freezing is accomplished by the rapid release and expansion of the cryogen (carbon dioxide) gas. There is a slim, Teflon-coated suction catheter that fits over the endoscope and is connected to the suction canister and built-in suction, which concurrently suctions the carbon dioxide gas while it is being administered. Hence, a nasogastric tube is not needed. The Polar Wand system has a smaller footprint and is portable.

EFFECTS OF CRYOTHERAPY

The immediate effect of cryotherapy is easily recognized as a white, sharply defined, frozen patch of tissue. After thawing, the tissue becomes engorged with blood and this can be seen as reddening of the mucosa and mild friability, possibly with some fresh heme. After 24 hours, the mucosal layer blisters and sheds. At 1 to 2 days, there may be cryotherapy injury seen as erosions and superficial ulceration. More than one session may be necessary depending on the size of the area and type of lesion being treated.

EQUIPMENT

- Same as for diagnostic EGD, except for the system-specific cryotherapy unit and packaged disposable catheter (through the scope) and suction catheter (Figure 6-32).

NURSING IMPLICATIONS

PREPROCEDURE

- Same as for diagnostic EGD, except for preparation of cryotherapy unit and specific cryogen delivery catheters and suction catheters, which should be set up according to the manufacturers' instructions.

INTRAPROCEDURE

- Same as for diagnostic EGD, except that the nurse should palpate the abdomen frequently for excessive distention and inform the physician so he or she can suction the excess gas. Excess gas in the stomach may compromise the patient's respiratory status. The cryogen dosing is based on seconds of spray (based upon the lesion being treated), which is tracked by the cryotherapy machine or a timer.

POSTPROCEDURE

- Same as for diagnostic EGD.
- If necessary make appointment for subsequent therapy.

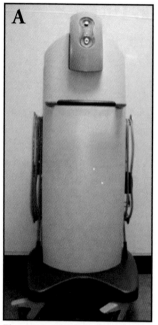 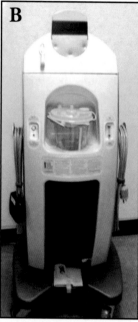

Figure 6-32. Polar Wand cryotherapy machine front (A) and back (B).

PHOTODYNAMIC THERAPY

Marcia Irene Canto, MD, MHS

Photodynamic therapy (PDT) refers to the use of photosensitizing pure red laser light to treat premalignant and malignant conditions, including those of the GI tract. It requires the IV administration of a photosensitizing drug (most commonly used, porfimer sodium; Photofrin, Pinnacle Biologics) followed 40 to 50 hours later by the endoscopic application of low-level laser light to selectively destroy dysplastic tissue. A laser fiber inserted through the biopsy channel of the endoscope is positioned next to the target lesion or mucosa, or in the bile duct (for malignant strictures, such as cholangiocarcinoma) to selectively destroy cancer cells while limiting damage to surrounding tissue. The course of treatment may require several applications (Figure 6-33).

EQUIPMENT FOR PHOTOFRIN INJECTION
- IV supplies (angiocatheter, heparin lock)
- Scale to measure patient's weight to calculate drug dosage
- Photofrin
- Towel (to protect the injection site from light)

NURSING IMPLICATIONS FOR PORFIMER SODIUM INJECTION

The patient is scheduled for a visit 2 days before the planned laser treatment session (eg, Monday) for IV administration of the photosensitizing drug (porfimer sodium). Prior to this visit, the patient must have undergone counseling and education regarding the possible side effects of the photosensitizing drug (sunburn reaction, in particular) and dietary changes. The patient should come to this visit already prepared with sunglasses, hat, long-sleeved shirt, pants, gloves, and other clothing that will completely protect skin and eyes from visible light exposure. The nurse typically also sends written information and instructions to the patient and reviews these in advance to confirm understanding and preparation.

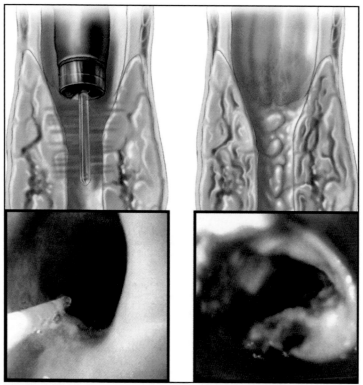

Figure 6-33. Endoscopic technique of light application with subsequent tumor destruction.

PREPROCEDURE (2 DAYS BEFORE THE SCHEDULED ENDOSCOPY VISIT)

- Verify allergies.
- Document vital signs and oxygen saturation.
- Make sure the patient has an understanding of the adverse effects of Photofrin, including light sensitivity.
- The nurse should confirm prior to injection that the diode laser is working, that the drug is available for injection, and the appropriate protective clothing are available.
- Check for appropriate protective clothing to keep the patient completely shielded from the sun.
- Insert an IV catheter with heparin lock adapter. Confirm proper placement of the catheter via blood aspiration and free injection of saline without extravasation.

- Weigh the patient.
- The physician should obtain an informed consent from the patient or responsible adult.
- The physician must provide an order for porfimer sodium injection with dose 2 mg/kg slow IV push over 3 to 5 minutes. Secure the medication and verify the calculation of dosage with another nurse. Always check the Photofrin package insert for precautions, contraindications, and recommended dosage prior to administration.

POSTPROCEDURE

- The patient should remain in the recovery room for at least 30 minutes to watch for any untoward drug reactions.
- The patient must leave the area with sunglasses and protective clothing.
- The patient returns 2 days after injection of porfimer sodium (typically on a Wednesday).

INTRAPROCEDURE

Equipment needed for PDT (Figure 6-34):
- Endoscope
- Bite block
- Topical anesthetic
- Water bottle
- 630 PDT diode laser
- Delivery fiber (different lengths available, typically with diffuser length of 10 to 25 mm are used)
- Inner cuvette for calibration
- Safety glasses for patient and staff
- Laser "Warning" sign for entrance into procedure room
- The patient should arrive with protective clothing and sunglasses.
- The patient should be prepared for an EGD.
- The diode laser should be turned on and calibrated according to manufacturer instructions.

The fiberoptic for laser administration should be selected by the physician, depending upon the treatment indication. The dose for the laser light is typically already programmed into the diode laser standard settings (selected by the physician), or the physician may select a custom energy (power) setting and time. The light dosimetry for advanced esophageal cancer is higher (300 joules/cm, or about 750 seconds of laser light using a 2.5 cm fiber) compared to Barrett's esophagus (180 to 250 joules/cm).

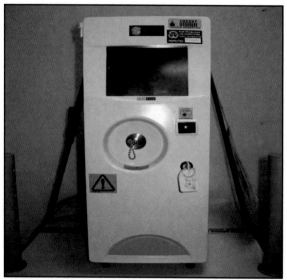

Figure 6-34. PDT module.

The diode laser counts down from the programmed number of seconds of laser light to be applied. The nurse will turn the diode laser light on and off as the physician holds the fiber and scope in place to optimize application of light to the target area.

After the entire amount (time) of laser light has been applied, the fiber must be wiped down with alcohol and stored with the patient's information on the box so that it can be reused, if needed at the following endoscopy visit.

POSTPROCEDURE

The patient typically needs at least 1 L of saline to be given during the endoscopic visit. The patient must have reminders regarding increasing postoperative (PO) fluid intake, medications (Larry's solution, PO liquid oxycodone, acetaminophen), and modified diet.

The patient returns for a second endoscopy visit 2 days after the first photoirradiation session (typically on a Friday) to check the effects of the PDT. A shorter application of laser light may be applied for any visibly untreated (skip) areas, usually 50 seconds or less.

POSTPROCEDURE

- Upon patient discharge, the nurse should verify the patient is wearing protective clothing. The possible adverse effects of Photofrin may occur for up to 1 month. After this period of time, exposure to sunlight should be gradual.
- Patients should be advised to call their physician with signs of respiratory distress, itching, or anaphylaxis.
- The importance of staying well-hydrated (which may be difficult because of concomitant swallowing difficulties) should be emphasized to the patient. Clear to full-liquid diet is usually necessary throughout the treatment.

NURSING IMPLICATIONS FOR PDT TREATMENT

PREPROCEDURE

- Same as for a diagnostic EGD.
- The patient should be instructed about the following:
  - ▷ Photosensitivity precautions (eg, avoiding direct sunlight, wearing appropriate clothing, and eye coverings)
  - ▷ Importance of taking prescribed pain medications as necessary
  - ▷ Importance of adequate hydration
  - ▷ Importance of follow-up care

INTRAPROCEDURE

- Patient positioning: Same as for a diagnostic EGD.
- Patient monitoring: Same as for a diagnostic EGD.
- Topical anesthetic: Same as for a diagnostic EGD.
- Follow the manufacturer's instructions for setting up the 630 PDT Laser.
- Provide safety glasses for all staff and the patient.
- Additional comfort measures: Same as for a diagnostic EGD.

POSTPROCEDURE

- Same as for a diagnostic EGD.
- Discharge patients with instructions regarding protective clothing, diet (clear to full-liquid diet), prescriptions for pain, a premixed solution consisting of an antacid and antihistamine for throat discomfort, antiemetics, and a PPI.
- Home health care referral.

ENDOSCOPIC MUCOSAL RESECTION

Eun Ji Shin, MD

Endoscopic mucosal resection (EMR) refers to endoscopic removal of the GI mucosa. This technique is used to treat patients with dysplasia and early superficial cancer confined to the mucosa layer. The most common techniques of EMR are strip biopsy, double-snare polypectomy, and resection using a cap and the Cook Medical Duette Multi-Band Mucosectomy (Cook Medical Inc).

The following is an abbreviated explanation of each method:

- Strip biopsy: This method utilizes a double-channel endoscope with grasping forceps and a snare. The lesion border is marked with electrocautery. Using a sclerotherapy needle, saline is injected into the submucosa below the lesion, causing separation from the muscle layer and protrusion. Grasping forceps are then passed through the loop of a snare to elevate the tissue. The mucosa surrounding the lesion is then grasped and strangulated with the snare. The resection is accomplished with snare electrocautery (Figure 6-35).
- Double-snare polypectomy: This method uses a double-channel endoscope with two snares and is suitable for protruding lesions. The first snare is used to grasp and lift the lesion from the muscle layer while the second is used to complete the resection with electrocautery (Figure 6-36).
- Endoscopic resection by clear cap: This method utilizes a clear cap equipped with a pre-looped snare along the inside groove. After its insertion, the cap is placed on the lesion and the mucosa is aspirated into the cap. The mucosa is caught and strangulated by the snare and resected by electrocautery. The specimen is retained in the cap for histological examination (Figure 6-37).
- Duette Multi-Band Mucosectomy is a system that uses a combined multi-band ligator device and snare that allows simple ligation and snare resection of superficial lesions and early lesions and early cancers in the upper GI tract (Figure 6-38).

EQUIPMENT

- Same as for a diagnostic EGD.
- Double-channel therapeutic upper endoscope
- Sclerotherapy needle
- Washing catheter
- Two snares, one with electrocautery

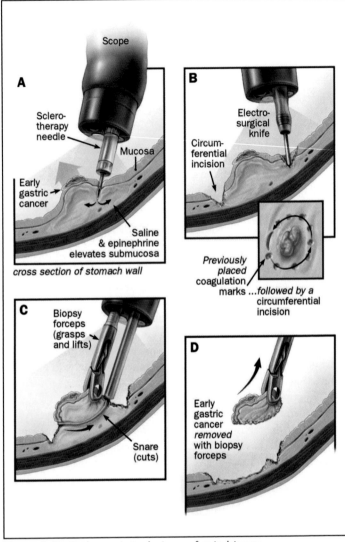

Figure 6-35. Endoscopic technique of strip biopsy.

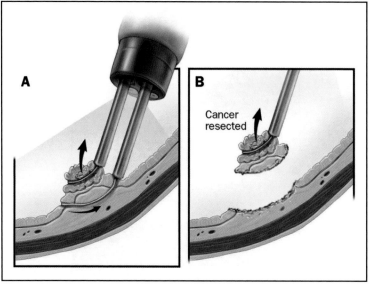

Figure 6-36. Endoscopic technique of double-snare polypectomy.

- Grasping forceps
- Needle knife with cautery
- Distal cap attachment
- Cook Medical Duette Kit

NURSING IMPLICATIONS

PREPROCEDURE
- Same as for a diagnostic EGD.
- Prophylactic antibiotics may be given at this time if appropriate.

INTRAPROCEDURE
- Patient positioning: Same as for a diagnostic EGD.
- Patient monitoring: Same as for a diagnostic EGD.
- Topical anesthetic: Same as for a diagnostic EGD.
- Additional comfort measures: Same as for a diagnostic EGD.
- During the procedure, the nurse assists in the injection of agents, such as saline.

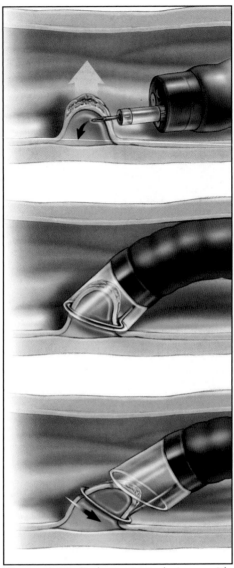

Figure 6-37. Endoscopic technique with clear cap resection.

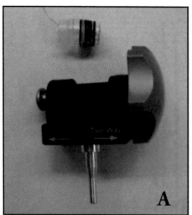

Figure 6-38. Duette handle (A) and snare (B).

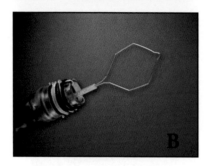

- If the patient complains of pain when the snare strangulates the lesion or if the nonlifting sign is present, endoscopic mucosal resection is contraindicated.

POSTPROCEDURE

- Same as for a diagnostic EGD.
- The patient should be advised to adhere to a soft diet for 24 hours after EMR to prevent mechanical abrasion to the excised area.
- The patient should be instructed to avoid any medications that may increase the risk of bleeding (eg, aspirin) for 1 week after the procedure on the direction of the physician.
- Vomiting, hypotension, chest or abdominal pain, or distention should be reported immediately to the physician.

Chapter 6

Laser Therapy in the GI Tract

Reem Sharaiha, MD, MSc and
Mouen A. Khashab, MD

Neodymium:yttrium-aluminum-garnet (Nd:YAG) laser has been used for the palliation of malignant tumors and for therapy of bleeding lesions. Laser therapy vaporizes tumors and coagulates bleeding lesions. Dilation may be required for obstructive tumors prior to laser therapy. The major complication of this therapy is perforation.

EQUIPMENT
- Same as for a diagnostic EGD.
- Nd:YAG laser unit (Figure 6-39)
- Laser fibers, cutter, and stripper (Figure 6-40)

Figure 6-39. Laser unit.

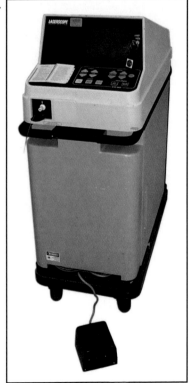

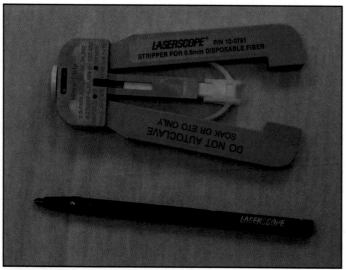

Figure 6-40. Laser cutter and stripper.

- Protective laser goggles for the patient and staff
- Charcoal filter to eliminate the escape of noxious gases during therapy (Figure 6-41)

Nursing Implications

Preprocedure

- Same as for a diagnostic EGD.
- If the patient is to receive prophylactic antibiotics, it should be done at this time.
- If the patient has coagulopathy, a recent prothrombin time (PT) and partial thromboplastin time (PTT) should be available.
- The patient should have NPO from midnight or 8 hours prior to the procedure.

Intraprocedure

- Patient positioning: Same as for a diagnostic EGD.
- Patient monitoring: Same as for a diagnostic EGD.
- Topical anesthetic: Same as for a diagnostic EGD.
- Additional comfort measures: Same as for a diagnostic EGD.

Figure 6-41. Charcoal filter connections.

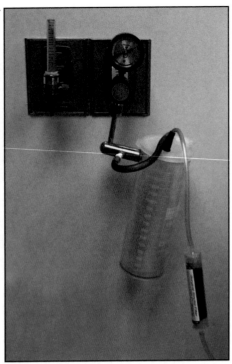

PROTECTIVE MEASURES

- Care must be taken to cover the patient's eyes.
- All personnel in the room should wear goggles, and a laser "Warning" sign should be posted above the door to the procedure room.
- The laser cutter and stripper may be used if the tip of the laser fiber may need to be cleaned or revised if deterioration of the fiber is noted during the procedure.
- If the fiber is removed from the endoscope at any time during the procedure (usually to clean or cut a new tip), the control panel should be switched to standby position to prevent accidental discharge.

POSTPROCEDURE

- Same as for a diagnostic EGD.
- Diet should consist of clear liquids for the first 24 hours, after that, diet can be advanced as tolerated.

Percutaneous Endoscopic Gastrostomy Tube Placement

David W. Victor III, MD

Percutaneous endoscopic gastrostomy (PEG) refers to the endoscopic placement of a semipermanent gastric feeding tube. The most common indication for PEG placement is failure of oral feedings. Patients with swallowing problems (stroke, severe psychomotor retardation, progressive degenerative diseases, neurologic neoplasm, or trauma) and patients with esophageal obstruction (oropharyngeal and esophageal carcinoma) may benefit from PEG placement. A PEG tube may be used to deliver unpalatable medications and supplemental feedings. PEGs are also used in patients for gastric decompression from chronic bowel obstruction or gastric atony.

PEG tube placement (Figure 6-42) can cause complications. The most common complication is from infection. More severe complications can include organ perforation or gastric leakage. Placement must be carefully considered in each patient.

Equipment

- Upper endoscope
- Bite block
- Topical anesthesia
- PEG kit contains skin cleansing swabs, sterile 4x4 pads, a vial anesthetic for injection, a 5-cc syringe with 25-gauge needle, 20-gauge 1.5-inch needle, a snare (pediatric endoscopes require pediatric snares), a scalpel, a 20-French gastrostomy tube with bumper and end plug, a fenestrated sterile drape, lubricant, and antibiotic ointment. Some kits also provide a hemostat and scissor.

Nursing Implications

Preprocedure

- Same as for a diagnostic EGD.
- The physician may prescribe antibiotics (usually a cephalosporin) to be given 1 hour prior to the procedure. This has been shown to significantly reduce infectious complications.

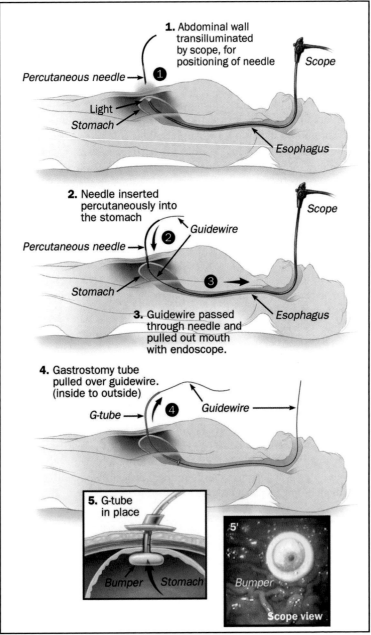

Figure 6-42. Steps of PEG placement.

- The patient or responsible caretaker should receive instructions regarding administration of tube feedings and care of the PEG.
- The room should be easily darkened to facilitate transillumination of the abdominal wall.

INTRAPROCEDURE

- Patient positioning:
  - ▷ The patient is usually placed supine with the head and chest elevated to about 30 to 45 degrees to prevent aspiration. This also exposes the abdominal area for ease of tube placement. When surveying the abdomen for proper tube placement, location of surgical scars should be noted. Scarred areas may make tube placement difficult.
- Patient monitoring: Same as for a diagnostic EGD.
- Topical anesthesia: Same as for a diagnostic EGD.
- Frequent suctioning is needed for increased oral secretions.
- Strict aseptic technique should be observed during the procedure.
- The nurse may assist the physician in transillumination (visualizing the endoscope light through the abdomen) to determine the site for PEG placement. This is best accomplished after the transilluminate light is enabled on the endoscope processor.
- Additional comfort measures: Same as for a diagnostic EGD.
- After the gastric tube is in place and the bumper is applied, care must be taken to ensure that there is no excess traction. This excess traction may cause a necrotizing fasciitis (necrosis of tissue under and around the bumper because of ischemia).
- Antibiotic ointment may be applied to the wound site.

POSTPROCEDURE

- Same as for a diagnostic EGD.
- The patient may remain on his or her back with the head elevated or may lie on his or her side until fully awake.
- Dietary instructions; instructions regarding signs and symptoms of bleeding, perforation, infection; and follow-up should be given to the patient before he or she leaves the unit.
- The patient may be discharged with instructions regarding care of the tube and feeding administration.

Chapter 6

CARE OF THE PEG AND FEEDING TUBES

- The site may be checked every 4 hours for the first 24 hours for purulent or bloody discharge.
- The area around the tube may be cleansed with soap and water.
- If there is thin drainage from the incision site, a dressing may be applied below the bumper site.
- Tube feedings (bolus or continuous) may begin 24 hours after the PEG is placed. Medications can begin in 4 to 6 hours.
- Bolus feedings are accomplished with a 60-cc syringe (without the plunger), allowing gravity to deliver the liquid food into the tube.
- Continuous feedings are facilitated by use of a pump. The enteral feeding is poured into a bag and infused over a 24-hour period.
- After each feeding or medication administration, the tube should be flushed with 60 to 120 cc of water using the plunger for flushing to prevent clogging.
- The tube should be aspirated with a 60-cc syringe prior to feedings to check for residual food. If more than 50 cc is removed, then feeding should not be instituted and the physician should be notified.

Percutaneous Endoscopic Jejunostomy Tube Placement

Stuart K. Amateau, MD, PhD

Percutaneous endoscopic jejunostomy (PEJ) refers to the endoscopic placement of a feeding tube in the jejunum. This procedure is performed in patients with abnormal gastric emptying or severe gastroesophageal reflux with aspiration. Endoscopic jejunostomy tube placement may utilize gastrostomy access (transgastric jejunostomy) or occur through direct percutaneous access of the jejunum. This chapter describes the former. Direct PEJ is performed in a nearly identical fashion to percutaneous gastrostomy tube placement; however, it should only be performed by an expert proceduralist given the greater mobility and lack of standardized position of the jejunum, thereby increasing the risk of complications.

EQUIPMENT

- An existing PEG tube in the case of transgastric jejunostomy.
- Same as for a diagnostic EGD.
- Upper endoscope or pediatric endoscope
- One of any number of available PEJ kits. Importantly, the PEJ chosen should be designed to match the existing PEG, as mismatched combinations frequently malfunction soon after positioning. Each kit typically contains the adapter to fit into the PEG tube, a 9 to 12 French PEJ tube, and a PEJ tube end plug (depending upon the brand, contents of the kit may differ slightly). Unified transgastric jejunal tubes exist as well and may be utilized if preferred by the physician.
- Grasping forceps, endoclip, or snare to assist with jejunostomy tube positioning.
- Syringe (10 to 20 cc) to flush the tube with water after insertion to determine patency.

Chapter 6

Nursing Implications

Preprocedure

- Same as for a diagnostic EGD.
- IV cephalosporin may be prescribed if PEG is performed prior to PEJ.
- Review discharge instructions with the patient and family before sedation. The instructions should also include care of a PEG/PEJ and feeding administration.

Intraprocedure

- Patient positioning: Same as for PEG placement.
- Patient monitoring: Same as for PEG placement.
- Topical anesthetic: Same as for PEG placement.
- Additional comfort measures: Same as for PEG placement.
- During the EGD, the physician should shorten the gastric tube to the desired length. The jejunal tube is threaded into the stomach through the PEG tube until the physician can grasp the tip or attached loop of string using grasping forceps, snare, or endoclip.
- The tube is then positioned into the jejunum with or without a guidewire in place depending of the physician's preference. Care is then taken to release the tube from the chosen device without leading to malposition on withdrawal. If an endoclip was utilized, the physician may ask the nurse for assistance with deploying the clip onto the small bowel.
- If a unified transgastric tube is to be utilized, the existing gastrostomy tube must first be removed. Therefore this may only occur 6 weeks or greater after the initial PEG tube placement to ensure an intact gastrostomy tract. Once removed, the distal end of the device is inserted through the tract.
- The nurse must be careful not to thread the PEJ tube (J-tube) through the PEG tube (G-tube) too quickly, as it will loop in the stomach and prevent proper placement.
- Once the physician determines that proper placement is achieved, the endoscope is carefully withdrawn.
- The J-tube is flushed with water to ensure patency and the guidewire is removed if utilized.

POSTPROCEDURE

- Same as for PEG placement.

CARE OF THE PEG/PEJ AND TUBE FEEDING.

- It is important to flush the tube with 60 to 100 cc of water after every use to prevent clogging.
- Feeding may begin immediately after insertion.
- Depending on the type of G-tube placed, a wound dressing may not be necessary. Cleaning the area with soap and water and applying an antibiotic ointment is sufficient.
- The patient should be instructed to notify the physician if the G-tube site becomes inflamed, painful, or has a purulent discharge.

UGI

Endoscopic Nasoenteric Tube Placement

David W. Victor III, MD

Endoscopic nasoenteric tube placement refers to endoscopic placement of a nasal tube into the duodenum or jejunum for short-term therapy for feeding and suctioning. Depending upon the tube type, it may have a gastric port for drainage or lavage. Drawbacks of the nasoenteric tube include erosion of the nasal cartilage, esophagitis, aspiration, and patient discomfort.

Equipment
- Upper endoscope
- Bite block
- Topical anesthetic if needed
- Nasoenteric tube kit (Figure 6-43) contains one nasoenteric tube and guidewire, stylet for stiffening, plug, and adhesive fastener.
- Water-soluble lubricant
- Grasping forceps

Nursing Implications

Preprocedure
- Same as for a diagnostic EGD.
- Review discharge instructions, including care of the nasoenteric tube and tube feedings, with the patient or caregiver before sedation.

Intraprocedure
- Patient positioning: Same as for EGD.
- Patient monitoring: Same as for PEG tube placement.
- Topical anesthetic: Same as for a diagnostic EGD.

Method #1
- The nasoenteric tube is placed into the nose before or after the endoscope has already been passed into the stomach. The tube needs to be well-lubricated with anesthetic jelly or water-soluble lubricant.

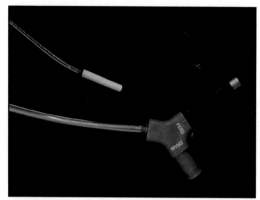

Figure 6-43. Nasoenteric tube kit.

- The physician grasps the string attached to the tube with grasping forceps and positions it into the second portion of the duodenum (fully extending the tube).
- The endoscope should be carefully removed and the tube flushed with water to ensure patency.
- The guidewire should be removed and the tube taped securely to the nose.

METHOD #2

- Other types of tubes can be inserted through the working channel of the endoscope and positioned through the scope into the second portion of the duodenum. The endoscopist will then remove the scope, leaving an oroenteric tube.
- The tube should be flushed and guidewire, if present, should be removed.
- This tube will need to be converted to a nasoenteric tube by attaching the end of the tube to a well-lubricated converter that has been placed through the nares and out of the mouth.
- The converter is then removed from the nose by pulling the orenteric tube up though the nares. Care must be taken to not dislodge the tube during this process.
- Additional comfort measures: Care must be taken not to pull the tube too close to the inside wall of the nostril, as this may cause ulceration.

EGD WITH ESOPHAGEAL STENT PLACEMENT

Reem Sharaiha, MD, MSc and Mouen A. Khashab, MD

An esophageal stent is an expandable metallic mesh or plastic silicone-coated tube used in patients with esophageal cancer for both palliative treatment of obstruction, strictures, perforations or fistula, and for benign indications. There are different types of stents that refer to the layer that coats the stent (fully covered, partially covered, fully uncovered [all metal] and polyflex [fully covered with polyester/silicone]). The advantage of partially or fully uncovered stents is that the uncovered parts reduce migration risk due to embedment, but it is more difficult to remove these, as the tissue grows through the uncovered mesh (tumor ingrowth or benign tissue hyperplasia). The stent can be deployed via direct endoscopic visualization and/or using fluoroscopy. The stent is advanced over a guide. If the luminal obstruction is not traversable by the endoscope, then fluoroscopic guidance is required. Dilation of the obstruction may be necessary before the stent can be placed, but should be avoided if the stent sheath can be passed without need for dilation. The stent then is advanced with the distal end beyond the area in question. Deployment should be slow, methodical, and with good communication between the endoscopists and assistant.

EQUIPMENT (FIGURE 6-44 AND 6-45)
- Same as for a diagnostic EGD.
- Guidewires (eg, Stiff or Savary)
- Expandable metal stents of different lengths and diameters (or Polyflex stents if deployment of a plastic stent is desired)
- Fluoroscopy

NURSING IMPLICATIONS

PREPROCEDURE
- Same as for a diagnostic EGD.
- Availability of stent sizes should be ascertained when the procedure is scheduled.
- The patient should be aware that severe gastroesophageal reflux might result if the stent is placed across the gastroesophageal junction.

UGI

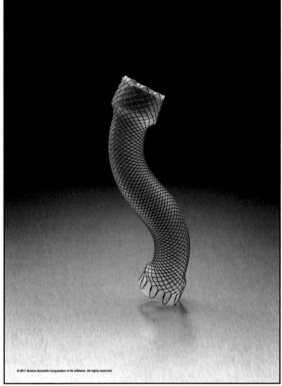

Figure 6-44. Fully-covered metal stent. (Reprinted with permission from Boston Scientific)

- The patient should also be aware that dysphagia may occur if the proximal end is close to the upper esophageal sphincter.

INTRAPROCEDURE

- Patient positioning: Patient should be in the supine position.
- Patient monitoring: Same as for a diagnostic EGD.
- Additional comfort measures: Same as for a diagnostic EGD.
- A second assistant is necessary to aid in equipment management and stent deployment.
- Fluoroscopy facilitates accurate placement of the stent.
- Radiopaque markers placed on the patient or contrast injected into the upper and lower borders of the tumor may be used as landmarks for stent placement.

UGI

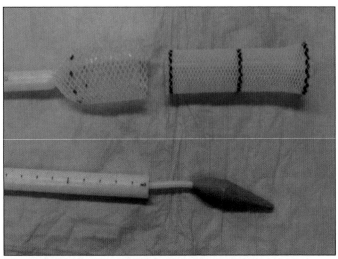

Figure 6-45. Silicone-coated flexible plastic stent.

- Oropharyngeal suctioning is important due to increased secretions (a result of esophageal obstruction) and concomitant risk of aspiration.

POSTPROCEDURE

- Same as for a diagnostic EGD.
- The patient may complain of chest pain following the procedure due to expansion of the stent. The patient should be evaluated by a physician for chest pain or abdominal pain following the procedure.
- Nutritional consult is necessary for patient education about a modified diet (eg, low-fiber, sips of water after each bite, sitting for 60 min after each meal).

PLACEMENT OF ENTERAL STENTS
Mouen A. Khashab, MD

Most enteric stents are made of an expandable metallic mesh and are used in patients with obstructive lesions of the esophagus, duodenum, jejunum, or colon. Enteric stent placement can be used for treatment purposes (eg, benign refractory esophageal strictures) or for palliative measures. The expandable enteric stent is advanced over a guidewire through the biopsy channel of the endoscope. Fluoroscopy may be required for the insertion of the expandable metal stent, especially when the lesion is not traversable with the endoscope. Dilation of the obstructed area should be avoided because of the potential perforation risk, but may be necessary before stent placement (Figure 6-46).

GENERAL PRINCIPLES

Two broad categories of stents exist currently: self-expandable metal stents (SEMS) and self-expandable plastic stents (SEPS). Semi-rigid plastic stents are no longer used.

Several manufacturers retail SEMS designed specifically for esophageal, duodenal, or colonic placement. These products differ in their physical properties and characteristics (length, diameter, flared endings, shortening during expansion, rigidity, material, radial expansive force, removability, and delivery systems).

Covered and uncovered SEMS are available. Covered SEMS are designed to resist tumor ingrowth, while uncovered SEMS imbed into the stricture and surrounding tissue. Fully covered SEMS may be removable, but have a higher incidence of migration. Uncovered SEMS are nonremovable, migrate less often, but tumor ingrowth occurs frequently.

One self-expandable plastic stent (Polyflex, Boston Scientific) is available for esophageal use. This stent does not imbed into the tissue and is approved by the US Food and Drug Administration (FDA) for benign disease and removability.

All self-expandable stents are able to be placed with high rates of technical success and often with fluoroscopic guidance (Figure 6-47).

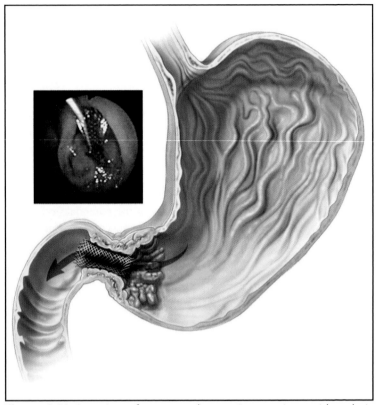

Figure 6-46. Location of an enteral stent in a patient with pyloric obstruction.

Equipment

- Upper endoscope or colonoscope
- Mouthpiece for upper endoscopy
- Dilators (Savary-Gilliard dilators or Balloon dilators)
- Guidewires (Savary-Gilliard guidewire or other .035-inch diameter guidewires)
- Expandable metallic stents of different lengths and diameters
- Fluoroscopy
- Water-soluble contrast
- Radiopaque markers
- Carbon dioxide insufflation (if available)

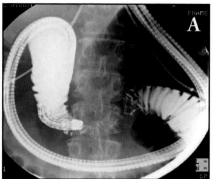

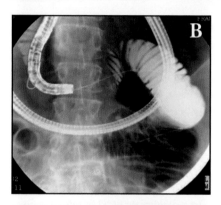

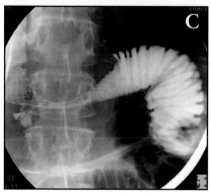

Figure 6-47. Endoscopic placement of duodenal stent. (A) Stricture is seen fluoroscopically in the third portion of the duodenum and could not be passed by the therapeutic gastroscope. (B) Wire is advanced through and (C) stent was deployed across the stricture.

Nursing Implications

Preprocedure

- Same as for diagnostic EGD or diagnostic colonoscopy.
- Prophylactic antibiotics are usually not needed unless stent is being placed to treat GI leak.
- The availability of stent sizes should be ascertained as soon as the procedure is scheduled. Stents are relatively expensive and may not be routinely stocked on the unit.

Intraprocedure

- Same as for diagnostic EGD or diagnostic colonoscopy.
- Patient positioning
  - ▷ The patient should be positioned in the left lateral or supine position on the fluoroscopy table.
  - ▷ In order for the physician to approximate where the stent should be placed, radiopaque markers may be placed on the patient to be used as landmarks for stent placement, or alternatively, contrast may be injected into the upper and lower borders of the tumor.
  - ▷ The patient should preferably be turned supine when using fluoroscopy to optimize assessment of stent position.
- Patient monitoring: Same as for a diagnostic EGD or colonoscopy.
- Additional comfort measures: Same as for a diagnostic EGD or colonoscopy.

Postprocedure

- Same as for a diagnostic EGD or colonoscopy.

Endoscopic Ultrasonography

Anne Marie Lennon, MD

Endoscopic ultrasonography (EUS) uses high-frequency sound waves to image internal structures. Differing reflection signals are produced when sound waves are projected into the body and reflected, generating an image.

The EUS scope can visualize structures within 5 cm of the ultrasound probe. This includes the esophagus, mediastinum, heart, left lobe of the liver, stomach, pancreas, left adrenal gland, left kidney, and duodenum. The EUS scope can also be inserted through the rectum and can be used to assess lesions in the rectum and left colon. EUS can be used as a diagnostic or therapeutic tool. Common diagnostic indications for EUS include staging of cancers, assessment of submucosal lesion, and assessment of pancreatic and biliary disease. Therapeutic EUS is becoming more common. EUS can be used to obtain tissue, for example, for confirming a diagnosis of pancreatic cancer. It can also be used to drain collections such as pseudocysts and to insert stents into the bile or pancreatic ducts.

There are three types of endoscopes: radial, linear array, and miniprobes. The radial and miniprobes produce images that are perpendicular to the axis of the scope, while the linear echoendocope produces an images that is parallel to the axis of the scope (Figure 6-48). The radial echoendoscope can only be used for diagnostic procedures. The linear echoendoscope is used for both diagnostic and therapeutic procedures such as ultrasound-guided biopsies (fine needle biopsy). Miniprobes are ultraslim ultrasound probes that can be placed through a therapeutic upper endoscope channel. These use higher frequencies to generate very detailed images of structures close to the probe. These can be used in obstructing esophageal tumors, in the bile duct, or to stage early cancers. The type of endoscope used is dictated by physician preference and the type of procedure being performed. The ultrasound endoscope is fragile and it is important to handle the tip gently. Ultrasound endoscopes should be hung in a closet with the tip encased in a plastic or sponge holder to prevent damage.

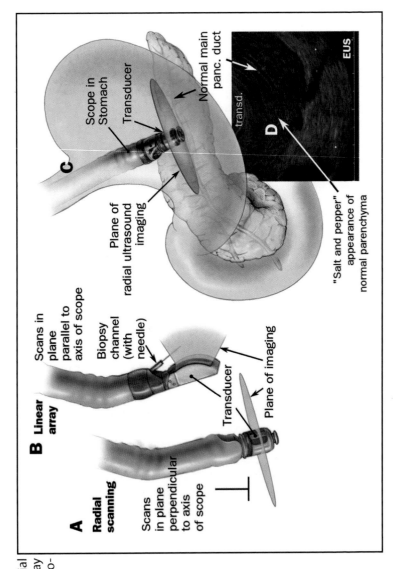

Figure 6-48. Radial (A) and linear (B) array ultrasound endo-scopes.

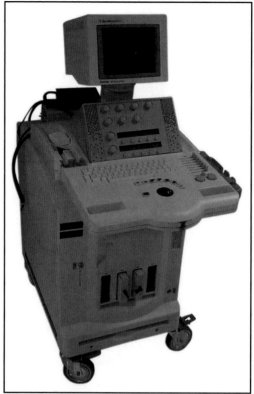

Figure 6-49. EUS unit.

EQUIPMENT

- Ultrasound unit (consisting of monitor, power source, and computer) (Figure 6-49)
- EUS endoscope:
  - ▷ The radial endoscope (Figure 6-50)
  - ▷ The linear array endoscope (see Figure 6-48)
  - ▷ Miniprobes
- Large water bottle with connecting tubing

Figure 6-50. Radial endoscope. (A) The handle of the echoendoscope and (B) the tip of the radial echoendoscope.

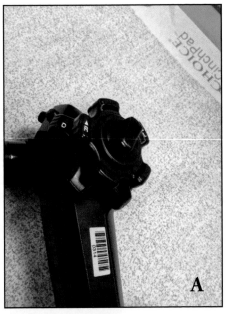

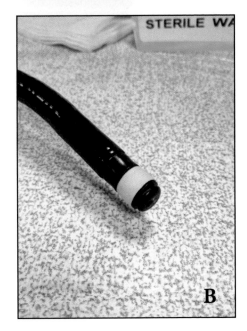

Nursing Implications

Preprocedure

- Same as for a diagnostic EGD.
- Ultrasound images cannot pass through air. Before placing the balloon on the endoscope tip, the nurse should make certain the balloon water channel is sufficiently purged to prevent the insufflation of large amounts of air.

Intraprocedure

- Patient positioning: Same as for a diagnostic EGD.
- Patient monitoring: Same as for a diagnostic EGD.
- Topical anesthesia: Same as for a diagnostic EGD.
- Additional comfort measures: Same as for a diagnostic EGD.
- The procedure may be lengthy; the nurse should keep the patient as comfortable and quiet as possible.

Postprocedure

- Same as for a diagnostic EGD.

EUS With Fine Needle Aspiration
Anne Marie Lennon, MD

Fine needle aspiration (FNA) allows the physician to obtain cells for cytopathological examination. The procedure is performed with a linear array echoendoscope. The lesion is located using the linear echoendoscope. Doppler ultrasound is used to insure that there are no vessels between the EUS scope and the lesion. An EUS needle is then passed through the biopsy channel of the endoscope and into the lesion to obtain cells. New EUS needles have been developed that can obtain a core of tissue rather than cells and are used if a large tissue sample is needed.

EQUIPMENT
- Same as for EUS
- FNA needle (Figure 6-51)
- Sheath
- Stylet
- 100 cc of sterile normal saline irrigating solution
- 10-cc luer-lock syringe
- Clear slides
- 95% alcohol

NURSING IMPLICATIONS

PREPROCEDURE
- Same as for a diagnostic EGD.
- Discontinuation of plavix 1 week prior and warfarin 5 days prior to the procedure.
- If the patient is to receive prophylactic antibiotics, it should be done at this time.
- If the patient has been on anticoagulant therapy, a recent PT and PTT should be available.
- A cytopathologist should be available at the time of EUS to prepare the slides for reading and interpretation.

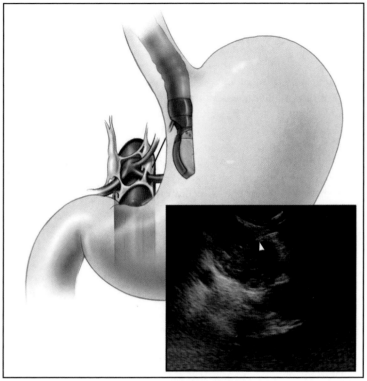

Figure 6-51. Linear EUS endoscope with FNA.

INTRAPROCEDURE

- Same as for EUS.
- An assistant is required for specimen collection while the nurse monitors sedation, patient comfort, and vital signs.
- An increased procedure time may be necessary since multiple (one to eight) passes may be required before an adequate number of cells are obtained.

POSTPROCEDURE

- Same as for EUS.

EUS-Guided Fiducial Placement
Eun Ji Shin, MD

Pancreatic adenocarcinoma is the fourth-leading cause of cancer deaths in the United States. Although surgical resection offers the best chance for long-term survival, unfortunately most patients present with advanced disease at the time of diagnosis. Chemotherapy and radiation therapy are therapeutic options in these patients. Radiation therapy offers loco-regional control of disease. Fiducials are gold markers that are placed within the tumor to allow a more precise delivery of high-dose radiation to the tumor, while limiting the radiation dose delivered to the nearby normal tissues.

EQUIPMENT
- Same as for EUS/FNA
- 19- or 22-gauge FNA needle (depending on the size of the fiducials used)
- Gold fiducial markers
- Forceps
- Bone wax
- Gown
- Gloves
- Drape
- Cart/table

PREPROCEDURE
- Same as for EUS.
- Cart/table should be set up with the drape covering the surface of the cart/table. The fiducial markers, bone wax, and FNA needle should be set up on the cart/table.
- Prophylactic antibiotics should be given.

INTRAPROCEDURE
- Patient positioning: Same as for EUS.
- Patient monitoring: Same as for EUS.
- Additional comfort measures: Same as for EUS.
- A physician or nurse assistant is required for the loading of the fiducial marker into the FNA needle.

POSTPROCEDURE

- Same as for EUS.
- Post procedural prophylactic antibiotics prescribed at the direction of the physician.

Chapter 6

ENDOSCOPIC PSEUDOCYST DRAINAGE

Vikesh K. Singh, MD, MSc

A pseudocyst is a collection of pancreatic fluid and small quantities of debris located within the pancreas or the peripancreatic tissues. It is distinguishable from a true pancreatic cyst because it is lined with granulation tissue as opposed to epithelial cells. Pseudocysts develop 4 to 6 weeks after an attack of acute pancreatitis when there is disruption of the pancreatic duct or its branches. Pseudocysts can also form in patients with chronic pancreatitis, trauma to the abdomen, or those who have undergone pancreatic surgery. Most pseudocysts spontaneously resolve and do not require drainage. Only pseudocysts that cause symptoms or become infected require drainage.

Abdominal imaging using either a CT or MRI/MRCP is required prior to the drainage of any pseudocyst. Imaging helps to determine the location of the pseudocyst in relation to the gastric or duodenal wall, the presence of debris within the pseudocyst, and whether the pseudocyst communicates with the main pancreatic duct. These findings help to determine the endoscopic drainage method.

There are two endoscopic options for drainage. The first is the transmural approach through the gastric or duodenal wall. A therapeutic upper endoscope, duodenoscope, or linear echoendoscope can be used for transmural drainage. The first two endoscopes require a visible bulge in the stomach or duodenum into which a needle knife papillotome is advanced. The advantage of using a linear echoendoscope is the ability to avoid puncturing a blood vessel or a varix when advancing a needle into the pseudocyst. Regardless of access technique, guidewire(s) are advanced into the pseudocyst under fluoroscopic guidance. The cystgastrostomy or cystduodenostomy tract is dilated using a controlled radial expansion (CRE) balloon between 8 to 15 mm. This is then followed by the insertion of one or more plastic or fully-covered metal stents.

The second technique is the transpapillary approach using a duodenoscope for ERCP. A pancreatogram is performed to identify the site of communication between the pancreatic duct and the pseudocyst. A pancreatic stent and/or nasopancreatic drain are inserted.

EQUIPMENT

- Linear echoendoscope, duodenoscope, or therapeutic endoscope for transmural drainage

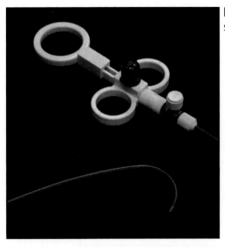

Figure 6-52. Needle-knife sphincterotome.

- Duodenoscope for transpapillary drainage
- Needle-knife sphincterotome if using a duodenoscope or therapeutic endoscope (Figure 6-52)
- 19-gauge fine needle aspiration needle if using linear echoendoscope
- Guidewires
- CRE balloon
- Double pigtail plastic and/or fully-covered metal stents

NURSING IMPLICATIONS

PREPROCEDURE
- Same as for ERCP.

INTRAPROCEDURE (FIGURE 6-53)
- Patient positioning: Supine.
- Patient monitoring: Same as for ERCP.
- Topical anesthetic: Same as for ERCP.
- Additional comfort measures: Same as for ERCP.

POSTPROCEDURE
- Same as for ERCP.
- Observe for signs of infection (fever, chills, abdominal pain) or hemorrhage (tachycardia, hypotension).

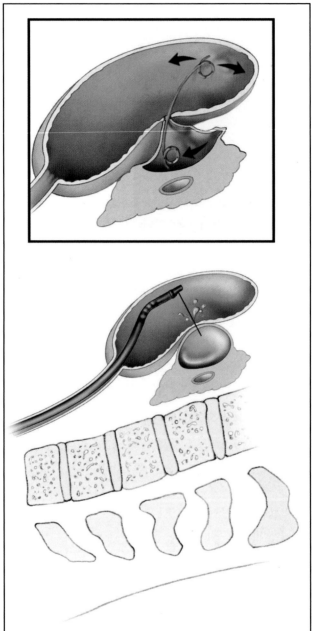

Figure 6-53. Endoscope technique for transgastric pseudocyst drainage.

DEEP ENTEROSCOPY

Gerard Aguila, RN, BSN and
Patrick I. Okolo III, MD, MPH

Small bowel endoscopy refers to endoscopic examination of the small intestine using any method, including wireless capsule and push enteroscopy. Device-assisted enteroscopy refers to specific endoscopic examination of the small intestine, utilizing an assistive device such as a balloon or spiral overtube. The term *device-assisted enteroscopy* may be interchangeably used to encompass all forms of deep enteroscopy. The procedures to be considered include the following:

- Spiral enteroscopy
- Balloon-assisted enteroscopy
  - ▷ Single-balloon enteroscopy
  - ▷ Double-balloon enteroscopy

The small bowel can be approached orally (anterograde) and frequently in a retrograde manner via the colon or an ostomy. The choice of a primary route often depends on the clinical situation. Deep enteroscopy is technically difficult and resource intensive. In most endoscopy units it should be considered a secondary or advanced skill. Deep enteroscopy is often a therapeutic procedure and so one has to have the required experience and skill base for interventions especially bleeding control.

TRAINING IN DEEP ENTEROSCOPY

Enteroscopy is performed in both ambulatory and inpatient settings. Most units will perform enteroscopy in the inpatient setting, so nurse training in enteroscopy is usually available only in the hospital setting. Deep enteroscopy is still relatively new, so team members including RNs may need to visit established centers to get training or to gather ideas about unit efficiency.

REASONS TO PERFORM DEEP ENTEROSCOPY

Enteroscopy is most often used in the setting of mid-GI bleeding. Mid-GI bleeding has been recently defined as bleeding from the ampulla of Vater to the ileocecal (IC) valve. This is in contrast to upper GI bleeding, which is now defined as bleeding from the upper esophageal sphincter to the ampulla of Vater.

Chapter 6

Obscure GI bleeding is defined as bleeding from the GI tract that persists or recurs without an obvious cause even after esophagogastroduodenoscopy (EGD), colonoscopy, and/or radiologic evaluation of the small bowel, such as a small bowel follow-through or enterocolysis. Obscure GI bleeding can be occult or overt based on whether or not there is macroscopic evidence of bleeding. The indications for deep enteroscopy include the following:

- Obscure GI bleeding
- Strictures of the small bowel
- Evaluation of inflammation, masses, and polyps
- To enable endoscopic retrograde cholangiopancreatography (ERCP) in situations where the intestinal anatomy has been surgically altered
- To place a direct percutaneous feeding tube distal to the pylorus (direct percutaneous endoscopic jejunostomy)
- To remove foreign bodies lodged in the small intestine

BOWEL PREPARATION FOR DEEP ENTEROSCOPY

Bowel preparation is not necessary for most patients undergoing enteroscopy by the anterograde approach. Patients should be ideally NPO for 10 hours prior to the procedure. In patients with profound motility disorders, a bowel prep can improve endoscopic visualization in the proximal small intestine. On the other hand, a complete bowel prep is necessary for all patients undergoing retrograde enteroscopy. A split dose preparation is ideal in these patients whenever possible.

EQUIPMENT FOR DEEP ENTEROSCOPY

Double-balloon enteroscopy was first described by Yamamoto in 2001. There are currently three different Fujinon (Saitama City, Saitama, Japan) double-balloon enteroscopes. The diagnostic enteroscope (EN450P5) has a 200-cm working length, a diameter of 8.5 mm, and an accessory channel of 2.2 mm. The therapeutic enteroscope (EN450T5) has a diameter of 9.4 mm and an accessory channel of 2.8 mm, making passage of accessories easier. The EC450BI5 has a working length of 1.52 and a 2.8-mm accessory channel. The shorter length of this double balloon enteroscope iteration allows the use of standard length ERCP accessories when this procedure is performed in patients with altered anatomy.

The Olympus single-balloon system has a 9.2-mm diameter high-resolution video endoscope, the Olympus SIF-Q180 (Olympus Optical). This endoscope is 2 meters long and has a 2.8-mm working channel.

Of note, spiral enteroscopy in its present form can be performed with any of these enteroscopes, with the exception of the EC450BI5 double balloon enteroscope.

OVERTUBES

The double balloon endoscope is accompanied by a 145-cm polyurethane overtube that has an inflatable latex balloon. The inner surface of this tube is lubricated with water and the balloons on both the overtube and endoscope are controlled externally by a balloon controller. The overtube used in single-balloon enteroscopy is often referred to as the splinting tube. It is a 140-cm long tube made of silicone with an inner hydrophilic surface. There is a single balloon at the distal end of the overtube. The balloon is connected to an external balloon controller that allows for sequential inflation and deflation of the balloon.

The overtube used in spiral enteroscopy is 118-cm long and 48 French in diameter with a 21-cm raised helical element at its distal end. Clockwise rotation of the overtube fits to a dedicated 9.1- to 9.4-mm diameter enteroscopes. It permits pleating of the small bowel, resulting in advancement through the small intestine.

CARBON DIOXIDE INSUFFLATOR

Carbon dioxide (CO_2) insufflation has been shown to be technically useful in enteroscopy. It appears to facilitate the depth of insertion of the enteroscope can in the small bowel. Patients experience less bloating and cramping when CO_2 is used for enteroscopy. The RN should be very familiar with the carbon dioxide generator available in the endoscopy unit. The standard air delivery in the endoscopy must be shut off and the appropriate mode on the CO_2 generator activated. Personnel who are familiar with the cylinder and the regulators on these generators should be the only ones charged with changing/recharging these cylinders. This is important for safety and will reduce anxiety related to carbon dioxide cylinders during deep enteroscopy procedures.

ENDOSCOPIC ACCESSORIES

Standard accessories for colonoscopy will suffice for deep enteroscopy through any of the enteroscope platforms with a 2.8-mm channel. Special length accessories are necessary to perform ERCP during enteroscopy except with the shorter double-balloon enteroscope. The nurse/endoscopy assistant must be familiar with all the potentially useful accessories and how to successfully pass them through the enteroscope.

CHECK LIST FOR ENTEROSCOPY PERFORMED FOR REASONS OF BLEEDING

- Enteroscope
- Overtube-Spiral versus single balloon versus double balloon
- CO_2 generator
- Electrosurgical unit (preferably one capable of performing argon plasma coagulation)
- Hemoclips
- Injection catheter–standard sclerotherapy needle
- Tattoo material (saline, sterile India ink versus spot)

CHECK LIST FOR ENTEROSCOPY CASES PERFORMED FOR REASONS OTHER THAN BLEEDING

- Enteroscope
- Overtube-Spiral versus single balloon versus double balloon
- CO_2 generator
- Electrosurgical unit (for ERCP, polypectomy, and fistula closure cases)
- Hemoclips (in the event of complications)
- Snare (standard colonoscopy length), Roth retrieval nets and specimen traps (if polypectomy is contemplated)
- Special length ERCP cannula and balloon (especially in ERCP cases where the ampulla is still intact such as gastric bypass patients)
- Dilatation balloon (colonoscopy length) for ERCP and stricture dilatation cases
- Biliary stents (usually 7 French diameter)
- Enteral stents (when enteral stent placement is contemplated)

In all cases, it is essential for the nurse/endoscopy assistant to understand the goals of the case and to have all the potentially necessary accessories identified and available.

CONCLUSION

Deep enteroscopy is a rapidly evolving area of endoscopy. Deep endoscopic access to the small intestine is now possible with the advent of these platforms. These platforms require a significant investment in terms of time and other resources. Proper training to ensure competence and mastery of these techniques is necessary in order to optimize outcomes.

Mid Gut

CAPSULE ENDOSCOPY
Christina Ha, MD

Capsule endoscopy allows the physician to examine the mucosa of the small intestine with the use of a very small video camera, the size of a large vitamin pill, swallowed with a glass of water. The capsule travels through the intestines, via peristaltic waves, capturing pictures at a rate of 14 pictures per second. The images are captured via sensors placed on various points on the patient's abdomen and sent to a data recorder worn on the patient's belt. After 8 hours, the recorder is removed from the patient and then downloaded into a special program on the computer. The physician is able to view all the captured images on the computer and detect the presence of ulcers or bleeding. Capsule endoscopy is used for diagnosing diarrhea, obscure bleeding, and anemia of unknown origin. It is also sometimes used for surveillance of certain familial polyp syndromes.

Contraindications of capsule endoscopy are patient's having implantable electrical devices, suspected intestinal obstruction, esophageal swallowing disorders, or strictures.

EQUIPMENT
- Video capsule (Figure 6-54)
- Data recorder and belt
- Battery pack
- Chargers
- 8 electrodes
- RAPID (Reporting and processing of images and data) application and software package (Given Imaging Inc)
- Glass of water with a few drops of simethecone

NURSING IMPLICATIONS

PREPROCEDURE
- Charge the battery pack the evening before the procedure according to the manufacturer's instructions.
- The morning prior to the procedure, the patient may have a regular breakfast and then clear liquids until 10 pm.

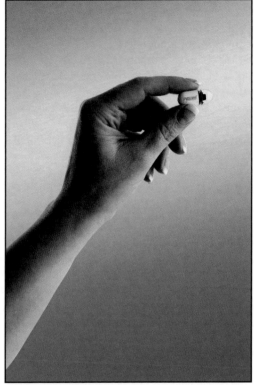

Figure 6-54. Video capsule.

- Patient should not eat or drink anything after 10 pm the night before the procedure, and should refrain from taking medication for 2 hours before the procedure.
- Instruct the patient to wear loose fitting clothing.
- If the patient has a hairy abdomen, instruct him or her to shave an area 6 inches above and 6 inches below the navel in a square.
- Early the morning of the procedure calibrate the electrodes and download the information into the recorder according to the manufacturer's instructions.
- Obtain the patient's height, weight, and waist size in inches. Also needed are a brief medical and surgical history, patient allergies, and a review of the contraindications with the patient.
- Informed consent should be obtained.

Chapter 6

INTRAPROCEDURE

- Attach the electrodes and data recorder to the patient as per the manufacturer's instructions.
- Videotape the patient's name and identifying information; also have patient hold video capsule up to his or her face to take a picture for identification purposes.
- Have patient swallow the video capsule with a glass of water containing a few drops of simethicone.
- Patient may leave the area but must return in 8 hours or when the video capsule exits the body.

POSTPROCEDURE

- Instruct the patient not to eat or drink anything for 2 hours after the ingestion of the video capsule. A light snack may be ingested after 4 hours. He or she may resume his or her regular diet after the test is complete.
- Inform the patient not to disconnect the belt or suspenders until after the test is finished and to avoid strenuous exercise and bending over while the test is in progress.
- Have the patient check the blinking light on the recorder every 15 minutes or so to see if the light is still blinking. If it is not, instruct the patient to return to the unit for further instructions.
- Patient must check all bowel movements while the test is in progress to see if the capsule has passed prematurely.
- Patient must return to the unit after 8 hours to have belt and recorder removed.
- If capsule does not pass within 3 to 4 days, the patient should notify his or her physician so an abdominal x-ray can be performed.

Diagnostic Sigmoidoscopy
Mouen A. Khashab, MD

Diagnostic sigmoidoscopy is the endoscopic examination of the anus, rectum, sigmoid, and descending colon. It is used to evaluate chronic diarrhea, fecal incontinence, ischemic colitis, lower GI hemorrhage; to differentiate between bacterial dysentery, ulcerative colitis, and Crohn's disease; and as an adjunct to colorectal cancer screening.

EQUIPMENT

- Video or fiberoptic flexible sigmoidoscope (Figure 6-55)
- Light source
- Water-soluble lubricant
- Biopsy forceps
- Formalin bottles and labels
- Specimen trap
- Viral culture tubes
- Water bottle

NURSING IMPLICATIONS

PREPROCEDURE
Bowel, Diet, and Drug Modifications

- Bowel cleansing:
  - ▷ Magnesium citrate should be taken at 4 pm the day prior to the test, followed by a clear liquid supper.
  - ▷ The patient should remain on clear liquids until after the test.
- One to 2 hours prior to the test, the patient should self-administer two Fleet (CB Fleet Co) enemas (or tap water enemas). Patients with diarrhea should not take enemas but should remain on clear liquids.
- No sedation is given for this exam unless the patient requests it. If sedation is given, the protocol for IV moderate sedation should be followed.

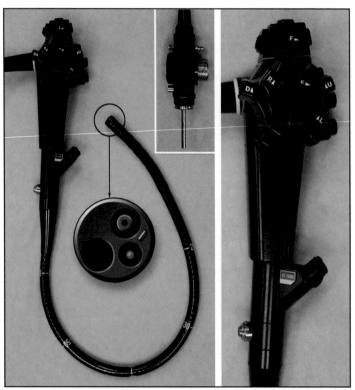

Figure 6-55. Flexible sigmoidoscope.

Endoscopy Unit

- The nurse will administer Fleet or tap water enemas if the patient was unable to self-administer.
- Baseline vital signs should be obtained including blood pressure, pulse, oxygen saturation, respirations, and pain level.
- Informed consent should be obtained.

Intraprocedure

- Patient positioning:
  - ▷ Patient is placed in the left lateral position with knees bent toward the chest.
  - ▷ Keep the patient covered with minimal exposure.

- Patient monitoring (performed if sedation is used):
  - ▷ EKG, blood pressure, and pulse oximetry should be monitored every 2 minutes while the initial dose of sedation is administered and then documented every 5 minutes unless the patient's condition warrants more frequent monitoring.
  - ▷ Suction should be readily available in case of vomiting from vasovagal stimulation or excess air retention.
  - ▷ Oxygen via nasal cannula at 2 L may be administered when using IV moderate sedation.
- Additional comfort measures:
  - ▷ Placing a pillow behind the patient's back and between the knees is helpful in keeping the patient on his or her side by lending support and reducing pressure between the knees.
  - ▷ Ongoing explanations of the procedure and visible images on the monitor may be helpful.
  - ▷ Soothing words of encouragement and light back massage may be helpful in providing emotional support.

POSTPROCEDURE

- All specimens should be labeled, bagged, and sent to the laboratory. Virology cultures should be sent to the laboratory within 1 hour of collection.
- Obtain vital signs including blood pressure, pulse, respirations, and pain level.
- If the patient did not receive sedation, he or she may be discharged with instructions (see Appendix 2) directly after the exam if vital signs are within normal limits and there are no signs of adverse reactions.
- If the patient was sedated, he or she should be kept on his or her side until fully awake and able to control secretions:
  - ▷ Monitor vital signs including blood pressure, pulse, respirations, oxygen saturation, pain level, and level of consciousness every 15 minutes (unless the patient's condition warrants more frequent monitoring) until they return to baseline.
  - ▷ The patient may be discharged home accompanied by an adult with discharge instructions (see Appendix 2).
- Patients undergoing screening flexible sigmoidoscopy receive instructions according to the findings of their exam.

DIAGNOSTIC COLONOSCOPY

Mouen A. Khashab, MD

Colonoscopy refers to the endoscopic examination of the large intestine (anus; rectum; sigmoid; descending, transverse, ascending colon; and rectum) (Figure 6-56).

EQUIPMENT

- Colonoscope
- Endoscopic light source
- Water bottle
- Colonic biopsy forceps
- Bottles of formalin
- Labels with patient's name
- Suction apparatus

ADDITIONAL EQUIPMENT THAT MAY BE NEEDED

- Cytology brushes
- Requisition forms and labeled containers for cytopathology
- Viral and fungal tubes for culture
- Mucus traps

NURSING IMPLICATIONS

PREPROCEDURE

Bowel, Diet, and Drug Modifications

- Prior to the procedure, the patient must undergo bowel cleansing:
  - ▷ Colonic lavage (GoLYTELY [Braintree Laboratories] or Colyte [Schwarz Pharma]) requires a shorter amount of patient preparation time (approximately 4 to 6 hours) but may not be well-tolerated.
  - ▷ Fleet phosphosoda kit (CB Fleet Co) requires a longer preparation time but may be better tolerated in some patients (should not be used in patients with impaired renal or cardiac function or the elderly).
  - ▷ Cleansing tap water enemas are an alternative requiring a clear liquid diet for 2 days for patients who cannot tolerate the oral method.

LGI

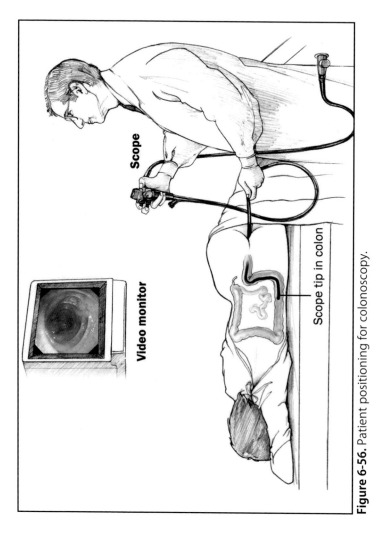

Figure 6-56. Patient positioning for colonoscopy.

- ▷ The nurse should be sure the patient has written instructions on the use of the bowel cleansing technique. If it is not possible to get written instructions to the patient in advance, a phone call with explicit instructions should be made several days prior to the test.
- The patient should refrain from using iron supplements (which may cause black staining of the bowel wall), aspirin, and NSAIDs 1 week prior to the procedure.
- Beets and red gelatin should be avoided 24 to 48 hours prior to colonoscopy, as they may cause a reddish hue to the bowel contents.
- Anticoagulant therapy such as Coumadin (warfarin sodium) or heparin should be discontinued prior to the procedure on the advice of the physician. Generally, Coumadin is discontinued 1 week before the procedure and heparin may be discontinued 4 hours before the procedure.
- Secure a responsible adult to accompany the patient home.

Endoscopy Unit

- Document baseline blood pressure, pulse, respirations, oxygen saturation, and pain level.
- Document medication allergies and daily medications with dose and frequency.
- The physician should obtain an informed consent from the patient or responsible adult.
- IV solution of D5/.45 NS or normal saline should be started.
- Discharge instructions should be read and signed by the patient or a responsible adult before sedation.

INTRAPROCEDURE

- Patient positioning:
  - ▷ The left lateral position with the knees bent toward the chest facilitates insertion of the endoscope and fosters the comfort and privacy of the patient. The patient may be rotated during the procedure to facilitate passage of the endoscope.
- Patient monitoring:
  - ▷ EKG, blood pressure, and pulse oximetry should be monitored every 2 minutes while administering the initial dose of sedation and then documented every 15 minutes during the procedure unless the patient's condition warrants more frequent monitoring.

▷ Vasovagal stimulation from excess air retention may cause belching and vomiting, therefore suction should be readily available.

▷ Oxygen via nasal cannula at 2 L may be administered when using IV moderate sedations.

- Nursing measures to facilitate passage of the colonoscope:

  ▷ The colonoscope may become looped during the course of colonoscopy. In this instance, the physician may require assistance from the nurse to apply abdominal pressure. Depending upon the area where the loop occurs, the physician will ask the nurse to exert flat pressure by using the palms of the hands. The loop often forms in the sigmoid colon, and by exerting flat pressure directly on the left lower quadrant, the endoscope may be advanced. This maneuver may be required at other points along the abdominal wall to facilitate endoscope passage.

  ▷ It is important not to apply excessive pressure to the patient's abdomen, as this may cause discomfort.

  ▷ If the physician is having difficulty advancing the endoscope to the cecum, it may be necessary to assist the patient in turning to a more supine, right side-down, or prone position.

  ▷ All specimens should be labeled, bagged, and sent to the laboratory. Virology cultures should be sent to the laboratory within 1 hour of collection.

- Additional comfort measures:

  ▷ Place a pillow behind the patient's back and between the knees to lend additional support and reduce pressure on the knees.

  ▷ Monitor vital signs for changes in pulse rate and blood pressure or expressions of verbal or nonverbal pain to keep the patient comfortable with IV medication.

  ▷ Soothing, calming words of encouragement along with light back massage may lessen the need for additional IV sedation.

  ▷ Try to maintain patient comfort and dignity at all times.

  ▷ The abdomen should be inspected and palpated frequently for distention; this may be alleviated by frequent suctioning via the endoscope.

LGI

Chapter 6

POSTPROCEDURE

- The patient should be kept on his or her side until fully awake and able to control secretions.
- Vital signs, blood pressure, pulse, oxygen saturation, level of consciousness, and pain level should be monitored and documented every 15 minutes until they return to baseline, unless the patient's condition warrants more frequent monitoring.
- Approaches for the patient having difficulty expelling excess gas:
  - ▷ Heat packs may be applied to the abdomen.
  - ▷ The patient may be encouraged to change position frequently or tilt the pelvis by placing a pillow under the pelvis.
  - ▷ Patients who are awake with stable vital signs may sit upright or be encouraged to ambulate.
  - ▷ The nurse may insert a rectal tube just inside the anal canal to facilitate passage of colonic gas.
- The patient may be discharged home accompanied by an adult with discharge instructions (see Appendix 2).
- The physician should be notified if the patient experiences abdominal pain, pain radiating to the left shoulder tip (Kehr's sign), bleeding from the rectum, or has significant changes in vital signs.
- The patient should be advised to avoid the use of aspirin or NSAIDs for several days after polyp removal, as directed by the physician.

CHROMOENDOSCOPY

Christina Ha, MD

Chromoendoscopy (Figure 6-57) involves the topical application of dyes to alter tissue appearance and improve localization, characterization, and diagnosis of dysplastic mucosal lesions (such as Barrett's esophagus or colon neoplasias). Chromoendoscopy usually adds 5 to 10 minutes to the endoscopic procedure.

Lugol's solution stains normal squamous cells of the esophagus brownish-black or greenish-brown within moments and gradually fades in a couple of hours. Abnormal cells do not stain. The technique is useful to detect high-grade dysplasia and early squamous cell cancers of the esophagus.

Methylene blue is avidly absorbed by the epithelial cells of the esophagus, small bowel, and colon. Dysplastic or cancerous tissue are less absorptive of the methylene blue dye and appear lightly stained or unstained against the background of darker blue stained normal epithelial tissue.

Indigo carmine is a contrast agent that is not absorbed by the epithelial cells of normal or dysplastic tissue. Rather, the purpose of the dye is to settle into the mucosal folds to allow for greater visualization and demarcation of potentially dysplastic pit patterns.

Acetic acid (vinegar) spray is used as a mucolytic agent and administered prior to application of the dye to enhance staining.

EQUIPMENT

- Spray catheter
- 60-cc syringes
- 20-cc syringe
- 30 cc of mucolytic solution (Mucomyst, AstraZeneca) (usually when using methylene blue for detection of Barrett's esophagus)
- 10 cc of 1% methylene blue
- 10 cc of 5% Lugol's solution (if requested)
- 10 cc of 1% to 5% indigo carmine solution (if requested)
- 10 cc of 5% acetic acid diluted with 10 cc of normal saline
- Standard endoscope or colonoscope (if routine biopsies are to be obtained) or therapeutic endoscope (if large biopsies are to be obtained)
- Standard or jumbo biopsy forceps

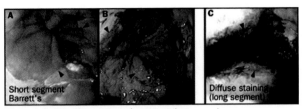

Figure 6-57. Chromoendoscopy (mucosa).

NURSING IMPLICATIONS

PREPROCEDURE

- Same as for a diagnostic EGD or colonoscopy.
- A recent PT and PTT should be available.
- If the patient is to receive prophylactic antibiotics, it should be done at this time.

INTRAPROCEDURE

- Patient positioning: Same as for a diagnostic EGD or colonoscopy.
- Patient monitoring: Same as for a diagnostic EGD or colonoscopy.
- Topical anesthesia: Same as for a diagnostic EGD.
- Additional comfort measures:
  ▷ Use a new biopsy cap to prevent dye from leaking out.
  ▷ Elevate the head of the bed to 30 degrees in addition to frequent oral suctioning to prevent aspiration during upper endoscopy.
- Acetic acid preparation:
  ▷ Put 10 cc 5% acetic acid mixed with 10 cc normal saline in a 20-cc syringe.
  ▷ Insert spray catheter through the biopsy channel of the endoscope and spray the affected area at physician's command.
- Methylene blue preparation procedure for upper endoscopy:
  ▷ Mix 30 cc of mucolytic solution with 30 cc of water in a 60-cc syringe.
  ▷ Mix 10 cc of methylene blue with 10 cc of water in a 20-cc syringe.
  ▷ Insert spray catheter through the biopsy channel of the endoscope.
- When instructed by the physician, spray the affected area with mucolytic solution and wait 2 minutes. When instructed by the physician, spray methylene blue and wait 2 minutes.

- Flush area with 60 cc or more of water until the area is cleared.
- Assist the physician with biopsies.
- After the procedure, flush the endoscope with 50 to 100 cc of water until clear of dye.
- Methylene blue preparation procedure for colonoscopy:
  - ▷ Mix 10 cc of 1% methylene blue solution with 90 cc of water to dilute methylene blue to 0.1% solution.
  - ▷ Fill 60-cc syringes with the diluted 0.1% methylene blue solution.
  - ▷ Insert spray catheter through the biopsy channel of the colonoscope.
  - ▷ When instructed by the physician spray the affected area with the methylene blue dye solution.
  - ▷ Assist the physician with biopsies.
  - ▷ After the procedure, flush the endoscope with 50 to 100 cc of water until clear of the dye.
- Indigo carmine preparation for colonoscopy: This technique is similar to the methylene blue dye chromoendoscopy for the colon.
  - ▷ Dilute the indigo carmine solution to 0.1% to 0.5% depending on the concentration of indigo carmine available (1% to 5%) using 10 cc of indigo carmine mixed with 90 cc of water.
  - ▷ Follow the same procedure for indigo carmine chromoendoscopy using the dye spray catheter as with methylene blue. This technique tends to be reserved for chromoendoscopy of the colon, not the upper GI tract.
- Lugol's solution preparation procedure:
  - ▷ Mix 30 cc of 5% Lugol's solution with 30 cc of water in a 60-cc syringe.
  - ▷ Insert spray catheter through the biopsy channel of the endoscope or colonoscope.
  - ▷ Spray the affected area.
  - ▷ After the procedure, flush the endoscope with 50 to 100 cc of water until clear of dye.

POSTPROCEDURE

- Same as for a diagnostic EGD or colonoscopy.
- It should be explained to the patient that his or her stools may be darker for up to 2 weeks due to the blue dye.

COLONOSCOPY FOR HEMOSTASIS

Mouen A. Khashab, MD

Colonoscopy for hemostasis may be performed to treat bleeding colon lesions such as bleeding neoplasms, arteriovenous malformations (AVMs), or other causes of bleeding in the colon.

EQUIPMENT

- Same as for a diagnostic colonoscopy
- Bipolar probe with energy unit
- Epinephrine 1:10,000 and saline for injection
- Sclerotherapy needle
- Clipping device
- Laser, APC, or cryotherapy unit

NURSING IMPLICATIONS

PREPROCEDURE

Bowel, Diet, and Drug Modifications

▷ Same as for a diagnostic colonoscopy, except in situations of emergent bleeding.
▷ Purge lavage (may require nasogastric tube).

Endoscopy Unit

- Same as for a diagnostic colonoscopy.

INTRAPROCEDURE

- Patient positioning: Same as for a diagnostic colonoscopy.
- Patient monitoring: Same as for a diagnostic colonoscopy.
- Nursing measures to facilitate passage of the colonoscope: Same as for a diagnostic colonoscopy.
- Additional comfort measures: Same as for a diagnostic colonoscopy.

POSTPROCEDURE

- Same as for a diagnostic colonoscopy.

LGI

COLONOSCOPY WITH POLYPECTOMY

Reem Sharaiha, MD, MSc and
Mouen A. Khashab, MD

LGI

Colonoscopy with polypectomy refers to the endoscopic removal of a colonic polyp using forceps or a snare with or without cautery, using an electrosurgical generator (eg, ERBE electrosurgical unit, Figure 6-58). A polyp can be removed en bloc or piecemeal depending on its size. If the polyp is small in size (<6 mm), it can be removed with biopsy forceps.

Once a large sessile polyp (≥20 mm) is visualized, saline mixed with indigo carmine is injected into the submucosal space to ensure lifting of the polyp. This is done for two reasons: to ensure that the polyp can be effectively resected (cancerous lesions do not lift), and to protect the colon from perforation postpolypectomy, as the lift ensures that only the mucosa is removed. After the saline lift, a snare is used for polyp removal. The electrosurgical unit settings are preset, but generally less power is used for right-sided colonic lesions as the colonic mucosa is thinner and can easily perforate. If flat portions of the polyp are unresected, these can be ablated using argon plasma coagulation. The polyp is subsequently retrieved with a Roth net or suctioned to be caught in the specimen trap. On occasion endoclips can be used to close polypectomy defects, especially in cases of deep resection or in patients who are at high risk for postpolypectomy hemorrhage (eg, patients on chronic anticoagulation).

EQUIPMENT

- Same as for a diagnostic colonoscopy
- Biopsy forceps
- ERBE electrosurgical unit (see Figure 6-58)
- Polypectomy snare, grounding pad, APC catheter, clipping device
- Looping device
- Sclerotherapy needle and epinephrine 1:10,000
- Saline mixed with Indigo carmine
- Specimen trap
- Polyp retrieval Roth net
- Container with formalin labeled with the patient's name or other identifying information
- Pathology requisition form
- India ink or GI spot for tattooing

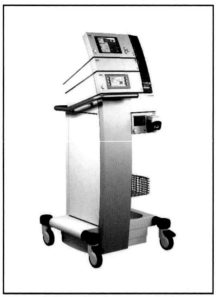

Figure 6-58. ERBE electrosurgical unit.

Nursing Implications

Preprocedure

Bowel, Diet, and Drug Modifications

- Same as for a diagnostic colonoscopy.

Endoscopy Unit

- Same as for a diagnostic colonoscopy.

Intraprocedure

- Patient positioning: Same as for a diagnostic colonoscopy.
- Patient monitoring: Same as for a diagnostic colonoscopy.

Postprocedure

- As per normal colonoscopy.
- Monitor for signs of bleeding or discomfort. Remember the larger the polyp removed, the higher the risk of perforation and bleeding.
- The patient should be advised to avoid the use of aspirin or NSAIDs for several days after polyp removal, if possible.

COLONOSCOPY WITH DILATION
Mouen A. Khashab, MD

Dilation of the colon is performed for strictures from surgery, obstructing tumors, and inflammatory bowel disease. Through-the-scope (TTS) balloons are most often used for these types of dilations. A colonoscopy is performed to the point of the stricture. At this point, a lubricated balloon is passed through the biopsy channel of the endoscope and advanced to the midpoint of the stricture. Fluoroscopy may be used to assist. The physician should direct the nurse to inflate the balloon while monitoring inflation pressure. The balloon is usually inflated for 1 minute. If necessary, the balloon may be reinflated several times. The physician may start with a small balloon and use increasingly larger balloons until the opening is large enough for passage of the endoscope.

EQUIPMENT
- Same as for a diagnostic colonoscopy
- TTS colonic or anastomotic balloon dilators
- Inflation syringe gauge assembly
- Sterile water to fill balloon (approximately 30 cc)
- Lubricant for balloon (vegetable oil spray)
- Fluoroscopy

NURSING IMPLICATIONS

PREPROCEDURE
Bowel, Diet, and Drug Modifications
- Same as for a diagnostic colonoscopy.
Endoscopy Unit
- Same as for a diagnostic colonoscopy.

INTRAPROCEDURE
- Patient positioning: Same as for a diagnostic colonoscopy.
- Patient monitoring: Same as for a diagnostic colonoscopy.
- Nursing measures to facilitate passage of the colonoscope: Same as for a diagnostic colonoscopy.

- Before handing the balloon dilator to the physician, the nurse should make sure it is well-lubricated with vegetable spray to facilitate passage through the biopsy channel of the colonoscope.
- Additional comfort measures: Same as for a diagnostic colonoscopy.

POSTPROCEDURE

- Same as for a diagnostic colonoscopy.

ANAL DILATION WITH HAGAR DILATORS
Mouen A. Khashab, MD

Hagar dilators are incremental metal sounds that are used to gradually dilate strictures of the anal canal (after ileoanal pull-through or other surgical or functional stricture of the anus). This may be done in conjunction with flexible sigmoidoscopy or by itself after digital rectal exam.

EQUIPMENT
- Hagar incremental dilators (Figure 6-59)
- Water-soluble lubricant
- Flexible sigmoidoscope

NURSING IMPLICATIONS

PREPROCEDURE

Bowel, Diet, and Drug Modifications
- No bowel preparation is necessary unless the physician is going to perform flexible sigmoidoscopy. If this is the case, preparation is the same as for diagnostic sigmoidoscopy.
- If sedation is not used, the patient may have a clear liquid supper at 4 pm. At 6 pm, the patient should take one bottle of magnesium citrate followed by two 8-oz glasses of water.
- The day of the procedure, two Fleet enemas may be self-administered 1 hour before arriving at the endoscopy unit.
- Patients unable to self-administer the Fleet enemas should arrive at the endoscopy unit at least 2 hours earlier so the nurse can administer them.
- The nurse should call the patient a day or two prior to the procedure to clarify the instructions and make adjustments as needed.

Endoscopy Unit
- If sedation is to be used, follow the same protocol for sedation as for diagnostic colonoscopy.
- Prophylactic antibiotics may be administered at this time if appropriate.
- If sedation is not used, baseline vital signs are taken before the procedure.

Figure 6-59. Hagar dilators.

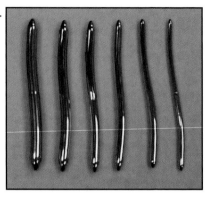

INTRAPROCEDURE

- Patient positioning: Same as for a diagnostic colonoscopy.
- Patient monitoring:
  - ▷ If sedation is used, monitoring is the same as for diagnostic colonoscopy.
  - ▷ If sedation is not used, no intraprocedure monitoring is necessary.
- Additional comfort measures:
  - ▷ If sedation is not used, the nurse will need to provide emotional support with calm, soothing words of encouragement and light back massage.
  - ▷ It is a good idea to have dilators and lubricant warmed (in a pan of warm water) before use.

POSTPROCEDURE

- If sedation is used, the procedure is the same as for a diagnostic colonoscopy.
- If sedation is not used:
  - ▷ Vital signs should be obtained at the end of the procedure.
  - ▷ The patient may be discharged as long as there are no untoward reactions, bleeding, or perforation.
- Warm-water baths may be recommended for patient comfort.
- The patient should be advised of the signs of infection and to watch for symptoms.
- Stool softeners may be beneficial to make bowel movements less painful.
- Patients should be advised to eat a high-fiber diet.

ENDOSCOPIC RETROGRADE CHOLANGIOPANCREATOGRAPHY

Stuart K. Amateau, MD, PhD
Mouen A. Khashab, MD

Endoscopic retrograde cholangiopancreatography (ERCP) is an endoscopic procedure in which the biliary and/or pancreatic ductal systems are visualized under fluoroscopy by injection of radiopaque contrast. ERCP is used to diagnose, evaluate, and treat biliary disorders including obstructive gallstone disease, inflammatory and malignant strictures, sphincter of Oddi dysfunction, and leaks. ERCP is also used to assess pancreatic ductal anatomy prior to operative, radiologic, or endoscopic intervention for chronic pancreatitis, suspected pancreatic trauma, pseudocyst, and aberrant anatomy among other disorders.

ERCP

EQUIPMENT

- Side-viewing endoscope (duodenoscope) (Figure 6-60)
- Bite block
- Light source
- Water bottle
- Wall suction, liner, and suction tubing with mouth suction
- Emesis basin
- 4x4 gauze pads
- Water-soluble lubricant
- Ionic contrast agent and 10-cc syringes
- ERCP cannulation and/or sphincterotomy device (various types, each with different characteristics; check physician preference prior to each case)
- Guidewire (various types each with different characteristics; check physician preference prior to each case)
- Electrical grounding pad for possible sphincterotomy
- Lead aprons and thyroid shields
- Fluoroscopy equipment

ADDITIONAL EQUIPMENT THAT MAY BE NEEDED

- Biopsy forceps long enough to fit through a duodenoscope
- Biliary cytology brushes
- Occlusion balloon
- Stone extraction device

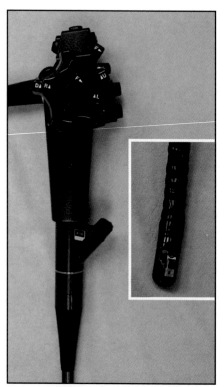

Figure 6-60. Duodenoscope. Inset demonstrates the head of the instrument.

- Specimen bottles with formalin
- Washing catheters
- 10-cc syringes for aspirating bile or pancreatic fluid

NURSING IMPLICATIONS

PREPROCEDURE

- The patient should have NPO for 8 hours prior to the procedure.
- The physician should obtain an informed consent.
- Discharge instructions should be read and signed by the patient or responsible adult before sedation (see Appendix 2).
- Secure a responsible adult to accompany the patient home.
- Monitor baseline vital signs, including blood pressure, pulse, respirations, pain level, and oxygen saturation.

ERCP

- Medication allergies and daily medications, including dose and frequency, should be documented.
- The physician should be notified of drug allergies.
- Depending upon the severity of the allergy, steroids or an anti-histamine may be prescribed before the procedure. Nonionic dye should be used in this subgroup of patients.
- IV access with either D5 1/2 NS or 0.9% NS should be in place.
- Prophylactic antibiotics may be given at this time (if appropriate).

Intraprocedure

- Patient positioning (Figure 6-61):
  - ▷ The patient should be placed in the semi-left lateral position with his or her left arm behind the back and the right arm in a saluting position (during the procedure the patient may be moved to a fully prone position to facilitate ductal cannulation).
  - ▷ Secure proper body alignment to prevent nerve damage to extremities (this may require the use of an arm guard or body wedge).
- Patient monitoring:
  - ▷ EKG, blood pressure, and pulse oximetry should be performed and documented every 2 minutes during the initial induction of sedation, then every 15 minutes unless the patient's condition warrants more frequent monitoring.
- Emergency equipment, including suction, oxygen, and crash cart, must be readily available.
- Topical anesthesia: Viscous lidocaine swish and swallow or 4% lidocaine spray may be used to facilitate insertion of the endoscope.
- Additional comfort measures:
  - ▷ Frequent suctioning is important to keep the patient comfortable and the airway clear.
  - ▷ A wedge may be placed under the patient's chest to provide support while he or she is positioned on his or her side.
  - ▷ Patients may feel claustrophobic and uncomfortable; supportive nursing care is extremely important in consoling the patient and obtaining cooperation.
- Flush a standard ERCP catheter with dye before the procedure begins, ensuring absence of air bubbles.
- It is important to keep the catheter free of air bubbles because they interfere with the diagnosis of stones. When looking for stones, it is best to use half-strength dye (50 cc of dye with 50 cc of sterile water)

ERCP

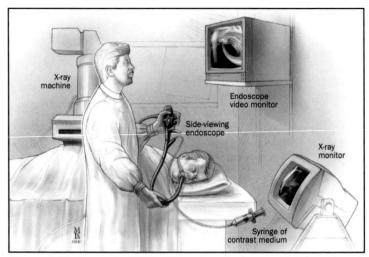

Figure 6-61. Set-up for ERCP with patient in the semi-left lateral position.

for easier visualization. Otherwise, full-strength contrast should be utilized.

- When the physician has determined the placement of the catheter in the bile or pancreatic duct, he or she may ask the nurse to inject the dye:
  - ▷ Gentle injection pressure should be used when infusing contrast to decrease the risk of pancreatitis.
  - ▷ A 10-cc syringe is commonly used because smaller-size syringes generate greater forces.
  - ▷ Patients who have been on narcotics for long periods of time are often resistant to sedation. If sufficient medication has been administered and the patient is still not comfortable, the procedure should be terminated and other forms of sedation used, such as propofol (an anesthetic agent). Propofol use is not considered moderate sedation and should only be administered by a physician licensed to do so.
- Upon access of the duct and determination of the disease state, any number of interventions may be performed such as sphincterotomy, stone extraction, dilation, manometry and stent placement (refer to associated chapters).

POSTPROCEDURE

- Keep the patient on his or her abdomen or side until fully awake and able to control secretions.
- Monitor vital signs, blood pressure, pulse, respirations, oxygen saturation, level of pain, and consciousness until the patient returns to baseline.
- Recovery after ERCP may be longer depending upon the amount of sedation used.
- Complications of ERCP include pancreatitis and perforation, which may be manifested by worsening abdominal pain, vomiting, fever, and chills. The physician should be notified if these complications are suspected.
- If the patient's recovery is uneventful, he or she may be released in the company of a responsible adult with discharge instructions (see Appendix 2).

ERCP

ERCP With Biliary Dilation

Anne Marie Lennon, MD

Biliary dilation is used to treat strictures caused by sclerosing cholangitis, bile duct injuries, or inoperable bile duct malignancies. Dilating balloons come in varying diameters. A sphincterotomy may be performed before the dilation (at the physicians' discretion). A guidewire is passed through the biopsy channel of a side-viewing duodenoscope and advanced to a point beyond the stricture. Once the balloon is placed across the stricture, a syringe filled with half-strength dye and a manometer is attached to the balloon port. The physician will direct the nurse to inflate the balloon to the desired pressure, usually for up to 1 minute. The procedure may be repeated until complete dilation of the duct is achieved.

EQUIPMENT

- Same as for ERCP with sphincterotomy.

ADDITIONAL EQUIPMENT THAT MAY BE NEEDED

- Therapeutic endoscope may be required (if larger than a 7 French stent is being placed)
- ERCP contrast dye and 20-cc syringes
- Guidewires (physician's discretion)
- Various sizes of biliary plastic and expandable metal stents (physician's discretion)

NURSING IMPLICATIONS

PREPROCEDURE

- Same as for ERCP with sphincterotomy.

INTRAPROCEDURE

- Patient positioning: Same as for ERCP with sphincterotomy.
- Patient monitoring: Same as for ERCP with sphincterotomy.
- Topical anesthetic: Same as for ERCP with sphincterotomy.
- Additional comfort measures: Same as ERCP with sphincterotomy.

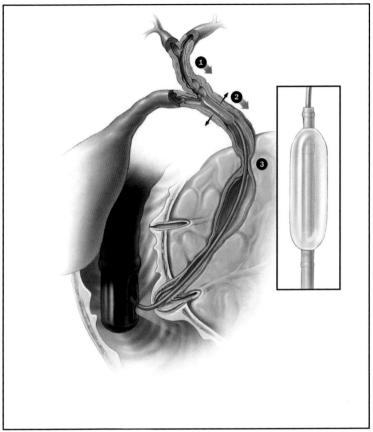

ERCP

Figure 6-62. Endoscopic technique of stricture dilation with dilating balloon.

- It is important for the nurse to have different sizes of biliary balloons close at hand; balloon size is determined after the physician assesses the size of the stricture on x-ray.
- It is not necessary to inflate the balloons prior to use because once inflated, the low profile is lost, making it more difficult to advanc- through strictures. The sphincterotome will be removed and the di- lating balloon will be threaded over the guidewire and pushed into position (Figure 6-62).

POSTPROCEDURE

- Same as for ERCP with sphincterotomy.

ERCP With Sphincterotomy
Anne Marie Lennon, MD

A sphincterotomy is an incision made into the sphincter of Oddi. It can be made into the bile duct (biliary sphincterotomy) or pancreatic duct (pancreatic sphincterotomy). A sphincterotomy allows greater ease of access to the ducts, which is important when therapeutic procedures are being performed, such as removal of biliary or pancreatic duct stones or dilation of a stricture. It can also be used to treat certain diseases such as papillary stenosis or sphincter of Oddi dysfunction.

An ERCP is performed to visualize the pancreatic or biliary ducts. The sphincterotomy is performed by inserting an endoscopic sphincterotome into the biopsy channel of a side-viewing duodenoscope. The sphincterotome is advanced into the papilla and strategically placed within the sphincter. During the procedure, the patient is grounded and the sphincterotome is connected to a cautery unit. The physician determines the cautery unit settings. Once the sphincterotomy is performed, the patient is ready for stone removal, stent placement, or dilation of the ducts.

Equipment
- Duodenoscope (a therapeutic duodenoscope is used unless there is a tight stricture or the procedure is being performed in a child. If using a diagnostic duodenoscope stents larger than 7 French cannot be passed through the biopsy channel)
- Light source
- Water bottle
- 4x4 gauze pads
- Sphincterotome with activator cord (Figure 6-63)
- Grounding pad
- Electrosurgical cautery unit with foot pedal
- Contrast medium and 20-cc syringes
- Guidewires
- 60-cc syringe with sterile water for flushing catheters and sphincterotomes

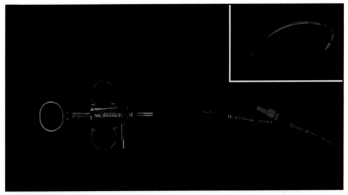

Figure 6-63. Sphincterotome.

ADDITIONAL EQUIPMENT THAT MAY BE NEEDED

- Epinephrine diluted to 1:10,000 if bleeding occurs
- Various stone-removal balloons used for tamponade in the case of bleeding
- Various extraction baskets

NURSING IMPLICATIONS

PREPROCEDURE

- Same as for ERCP.
- Medications that alter the bleeding time (eg, anticoagulants) should be discontinued on the physician's order for 1 week prior to the procedure.
- The physician may order an antibiotic to be given intravenously 1 hour before the procedure, if appropriate.
- The patient should have recent coagulation studies.
- It may be necessary to admit the patient after the procedure; preplanning for admission may be necessary.

INTRAPROCEDURE

- Patient positioning: Same as for ERCP.
- Patient monitoring: Same as for ERCP.
- Topical anesthetic: Same as for ERCP.
- Additional comfort measures: Same as for ERCP.

- The patient must be grounded to prevent burns occurring during sphincterotomy. Most modern cautery units will not function unless the grounding pad is properly placed and attached.
- Flush the papillotome with 2 cc of contrast dye and/or load with a guidewire (physicians' preference).
- It is the nurse's or assistant's responsibility to assist the physician in the manipulation of the sphincterotome.
- If a double lumen sphincterotome is being used, once dye is injected through the sphincterotome, flush the channel with sterile water before inserting a guidewire.
- If excessive bleeding occurs after sphincterotomy, the physician may request epinephrine diluted to 1:10,000 flushed through a sclerotherapy needle or injected around the bleeding site. Sometimes tamponade may be accomplished by using an inflated stone retrieval balloon pressed against the bleeding site.

POSTPROCEDURE

- Same as for ERCP.
- The physician should advise the patient about the resumption of anticoagulants.

ERCP With Stent Placement

Anne Marie Lennon, MD

Stents may be placed in the bile or pancreatic duct, most commonly to maintain luminal patency. They may also be used for dilation of strictures, to treat bile and pancreatic duct leaks, and to treat pancreatic pseudocysts. Stents come in a variety of lengths and can be made of plastic or metal. There is a variety of plastic stents, including straight, nasobiliary, or double pigtail stents that may be inserted into the bile or pancreatic duct. Metal stents can be uncovered, partially, or fully covered.

Equipment

- Same as for ERCP with sphincterotomy.
- Therapeutic duodenoscope is routinely used. If a diagnostic duodenoscope is used, stents larger than 7 French cannot be placed.
- Various sizes of plastic biliary and pancreatic stents, including expandable biliary stents or nasobiliary and pigtail stents, as requested by physician.
- Stents may be packaged as a kit and include stent, guidewire, pusher tubes, and catheters; additional stents may be purchased separately.

Additional Equipment That May Be Needed

- Dilating balloons or catheters
- Sclerotherapy needle
- Epinephrine diluted to 1:10,000 if bleeding occurs
- Various stone removal balloons used for tamponading bleeding (see equipment needed for ERCP with sphincterotomy)

Nursing Implications

Preprocedure

- Same as for ERCP with sphincterotomy.

Intraprocedure

- Patient positioning: Same as for ERCP with sphincterotomy.
- Patient monitoring: Same as for ERCP with sphincterotomy.
- Topical anesthetic: Same as for ERCP with sphincterotomy.

- Additional comfort measures: Same as for ERCP with sphincter-otomy.
- The physician will determine the size of the stent needed. If the stent being used is larger than 7 French, a larger channel or therapeutic side-viewing duodenoscope will be required.
- The nurse may be required to assist with wire exchanges during the procedure. The nurse will be responsible for maintaining the guide-wire position by applying steady forward pressure on the guidewire as the physician is withdrawing the ERCP cannula. Intermittent fluoroscopy may be used to confirm guidewire placement. The need for fluoroscopy is decreased when using marked guidewires.
- Stents larger than 7 French in diameter require the use of a guid-ing catheter. After the stent is threaded over the guiding catheter, a pusher tube may be used to advance the stent through the biopsy channel of the endoscope. The physician may request that the nurse place continuous backward pressure on the guidewire and guiding catheter. This will assist the passage of the stent over the guiding catheter and into the duct.
- Nasobiliary stent placement is performed directly over the guide-wire using a pusher tube to advance the stent. Once the stent has been positioned in the duct, it is externalized through the mouth and the endoscope is withdrawn. The nasobiliary tube is then re-routed through the nose for patient comfort. The tube must be se-curely taped to the patient's nose and neck (Figures 6-64 and 6-65).

POSTPROCEDURE

- Same as for ERCP with sphincterotomy.
- Drainage from the nasobiliary tube should be measured and docu-mented. Any change in color, volume, or odor should be reported to the physician.

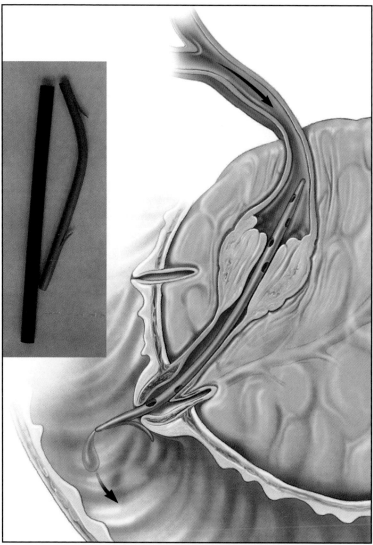

Figure 6-64. Plastic biliary stent across a tumor.

ERCP

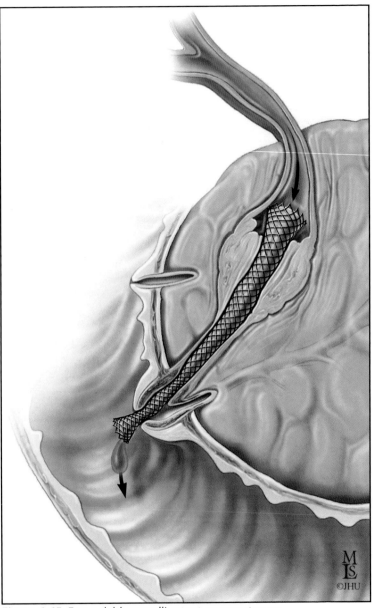

Figure 6-65. Expandable metallic stent across a tumor.

ERCP With Stone Removal

Vikesh K. Singh, MD, MSc

The removal of stone(s) from the bile and pancreatic ducts can be accomplished using a variety of accessories alone or in combination. The endoscopist may choose to use a stone retrieval balloon, a wire basket, and/or a mechanical lithotripter.

The removal of the majority of bile duct stones can be easily accomplished using a stone retrieval balloon. After the stone(s) is identified on cholangiogram, a biliary sphincterotomy is performed and a stone retrieval balloon is advanced to just above the level of the stone. The balloon (available in 8.5, 11.5, and 15 mm) is inflated to approximate the diameter of the bile duct and is gradually withdrawn, with or without concurrent contrast administration, and the stone(s) is extracted. This maneuver can be repeated until the bile duct is cleared of stones. There are occasions when the balloon has to be deflated to allow for withdrawal from the biliary orifice despite a prior sphincterotomy. The balloon can also rupture, particularly when stones have an uneven surface or are impacted.

The use of baskets and mechanical lithotripters are reserved primarily for the removal of larger and/or impacted bile duct stones. Both techniques require cholangiography to define the location, size, and number of stones. A biliary sphincterotomy must be performed to facilitate the passage of either device into the bile duct and to ensure that the biliary orifice can accommodate the removal of a stone. There are 4 and 8 wire baskets. The basket is inserted into the bile duct, advanced to a level above the stone(s), and opened. While withdrawing the basket from the duct it is usually closed and then removed with the stones grasped within the wires. If stones are retrieved, the basket is reopened and the stones are released into the duodenum and passed in the stool. This procedure can be repeated several times until all stones are removed.

Mechanical lithotripsy is usually reserved for large stone(s), typically measuring 12 to 20 mm in diameter, which cannot be removed using other techniques. A mechanical lithotripter (a basket-type instrument with stone crushing capability) is inserted into the bile duct and advanced to the level of the stone(s). A metal wire running from the basket through the biopsy channel of the duodenoscope is brought externally and affixed to a winding device. The winding device contracts the basket tightly around the stones. The basket contraction results in stone fragmentation. A stone retrieval balloon is then used to remove the smaller stone fragments into the duodenum.

Obstructing pancreatic duct stones can cause pain or acute recurrent pancreatitis in patients with chronic pancreatitis. These can be difficult to remove using the same techniques as bile duct stones since they are calcified and impacted against the pancreatic duct wall. After pancreatography defines the level of the obstructing stone(s), a stone retrieval balloon can be inserted and withdrawn, but this rarely results in successful removal and the balloon will often rupture against the calcified stone(s). Baskets and mechanical lithotripters are rarely used since the pancreatic duct diameter is often too narrow to allow for the appropriate opening of these devices within the duct. Most patients will require extracorporeal shockwave lithotripsy (ESWL) to fragment these stones prior to ERCP. ESWL is a technique where concentrated sound waves are applied externally to the abdomen to fragment pancreatic stones. Several sessions are often required to result in complete dissolution of the stones prior to ERCP.

EQUIPMENT
- Same as for ERCP with sphincterotomy.
- ESWL for pancreatic duct stones.

ADDITIONAL EQUIPMENT THAT MAY BE NEEDED
- Stone retrieval baskets (Figure 6-66)
- Stone retrieval balloons (Figure 6-67)
- Mechanical lithotripter (Figure 6-68)

NURSING IMPLICATIONS

PREPROCEDURE
- Same as for ERCP with sphincterotomy.

INTRAPROCEDURE
- Patient positioning: Same as for ERCP with sphincterotomy.
- Patient monitoring: Same as for ERCP with sphincterotomy.
- Topical anesthesia: Same as for ERCP with sphincterotomy.

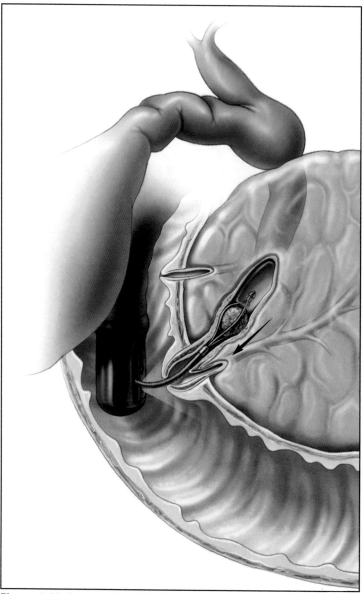

Figure 6-66. Stone retrieval basket.

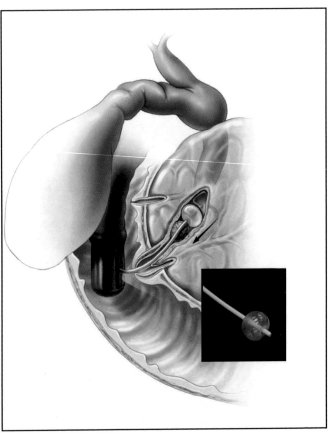

Figure 6-67. Stone retrieval balloon.

Figure 6-68. Endoscopic lithotriptor.

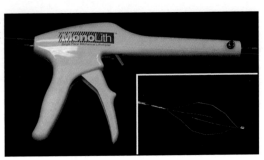

- Additional comfort measures: Same as for ERCP with sphincterotomy.
- If excessive bleeding occurs after sphincterotomy, the endoscopist may request epinephrine diluted to 1:10,000 or NS flushed through a sclerotherapy needle to be injected around the sphincterotomy incision site.
- Before the basket is inserted through the biopsy channel of the duodenoscope, the nurse should check to make sure the working parts are functioning properly. The endoscopist may decide to load the basket with a wire or flush it with dye before insertion.
- The endoscopist will direct the nurse to open the basket after it is advanced to a level above the stone(s). As the endoscopist pulls the basket back, he or she will direct the nurse to close it.
- The sphincterotome is removed over the guidewire or glidewire and the balloon or mechanical lithotripter is inserted. When the exchange begins, the responsibility of the nurse is to apply steady forward pressure to the guidewire as the physician is withdrawing the sphincterotome. This keeps the guidewire in position within the duct. Communication between nurse and endoscopist is essential for success.
- Intermittent fluoroscopy may be used to ensure the guidewire is in place (if marked guidewires are used, it lessens the need for fluoroscopy).
- The balloon should be inflated prior to insertion into the biopsy channel of the duodenoscope.
- The nurse will be instructed to inflate the balloon once it is positioned. The nurse should check the balloon specifications (on the packaging) to ensure the proper amount of air inflation. The endoscopist will direct the nurse to inflate or deflate the balloon as needed.
- The nurse should check with the endoscopist in advance to see if the mechanical lithotripter will be needed for stone fragmentation. It is the responsibility of the nurse to assemble it.

POSTPROCEDURE
- Same as for ERCP with sphincterotomy.

ERCP

CHOLANGIOSCOPY

Zhiping Li, MD and
David W. Victor III, MD

Cholangioscopy is direct visualization of the biliary tree. This can be managed in a variety of ways. It can be accomplished via direct cholangioscopy that places a small upper endoscope directly into the bile duct, which is extremely difficult. The other option that is more commonly used is mother-baby cholangioscope where a standard therapeutic duodenoscope (mother) is used to identify the bile duct and a smaller cholangioscope (baby) is inserted through the working channel of the mother scope into the bile duct. There are several types of baby scopes available. Some use digital imaging and provide excellent optics but require two endoscopists and only have two way deflection.

The more common system used today is the SpyGlass Direct Visualization System (Boston Scientific). It is advantageous in that it allows for a single operator to piggy back the duodenoscope to perform cholangioscopy. The SpyGlass System includes the disposable SpyScope Delivery Catheter (Boston Scientific) that has four direction movement unlike other "baby" scopes. It is introduced through a therapeutic duodenoscope with a minimum working channel diameter of 4.2 mm. The reusable SpyGlass Fiber Optic Probe (Boston Scientific) provides the light source and imaging. (Figure 6-69)

The system allows for direct visualization of the inside of the bile duct. This can help determine if a stricture is cancerous, help to break up large stones, and help direct the guidewire past difficult strictures. Tissue sampling is also possible using the disposable SpyBite Biopsy Forceps (Boston Scientific). (Figure 6-70)

EQUIPMENT (SAME AS FOR AN ERCP WITH SPHINCTEROTOMY)

- Adult duodenoscope
- Light source for ERCP scope
- Water bottle
- 4x4 gauze pads
- Variety of ERCP catheters
- Sphincterotome with activator cord
- Grounding pad

ERCP

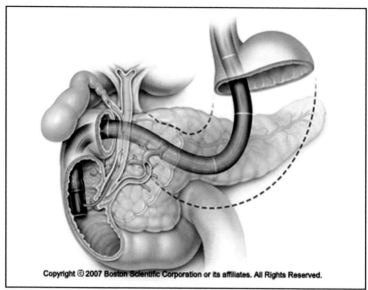

Figure 6-69. Spyglass cholangioscope delivered into the common bile duct via ERCP scope. The system is used after a standard ERCP and likely sphinterotomy has been performed and a wire has been placed into the bile duct. The system is advanced into the bile duct in a fashion similar to placing a biliary stent. (Reprinted with permission of Boston Scientific Corporation.)

- Electrosurgical cautery unit or argon plasma coagulator with foot pedal
- Contrast medium and 20-cc syringes
- Guidewires
- 60-cc syringes with sterile water for flushing catheters and sphincterotomes

ADDITIONAL EQUIPMENT FOR SPYGLASS SYSTEM

- SpyScope Delivery Catheter-Disposable (Figure 6-71)
- Fiber optic cable-reusable and delicate (Figure 6-72)
- Component cart and three-joint arm * (Figure 6-73)
- Light source and cable *
- Camera and camera head *
- Cord connecting probe and camera head *
- Power cord *
- Irrigation pump *

Figure 6-70. SpyBite Biopsy Forceps. (Reprinted with permission of Boston Scientific Corporation.)

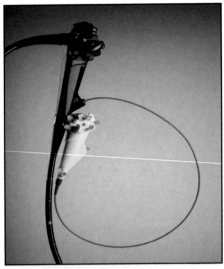

Figure 6-71. SpyScope Delivery Catheter. (Reprinted with permission of Boston Scientific Corporation.)

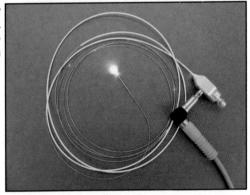

- Monitor *
- SpyBite Biopsy Forceps (see Figure 6-70)

*These items are typically contained on the SpyGlass Component Cart, which is shown in Figure 6-73.

NURSING IMPLICATIONS

PREPROCEDURE

- Same as for ERCP.

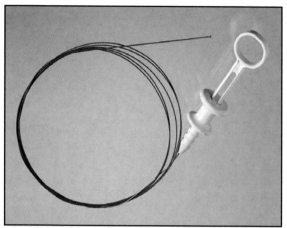

Figure 6-72. Fiber optic cable with light source adapter. (Reprinted with permission of Boston Scientific Corporation.)

- The physician may order an antibiotic to be given intravenously 1 hour before the procedure, if appropriate.
- The patient should have recent coagulation studies.
- It may be necessary to admit the patient after the procedure; preplanning for admission may be necessary.
- The unit should be checked for the previously mentioned components prior to beginning the ERCP.
- The camera unit should be cleaned and focused prior to beginning the ERCP.

INTRAPROCEDURE

- Patient positioning: Same as for ERCP.
- Patient monitoring: Same as for ERCP.
- Topical anesthetic: Same as for ERCP.
- Additional comfort measures: Same as for ERCP.
- The Nurse or assistant should open the disposable SpyScope Delivery Catheter when asked by the physician.
- The light source should be turned on and the fiber optic cable attached.
- The fiber optic cable should then be inserted in the clear plastic port on the head of the SpyScope Catheter and advance gently to the end of the SpyScope Catheter.
- The cable should be secure with a gentle right turn for tightening.

Figure 6-73. SpyGlass Component Cart and three-joint arm. (Reprinted with permission of Boston Scientific Corporation.)

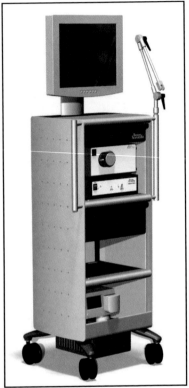

- The ERCP wire from the duodenoscope should then be back loaded though the biopsy channel at the end of the SpyScope Catheter.
- The SpyScope Catheter head should then be lashed tightly to the bottom of the duodenoscope with the clear plastic brace on the SpyScope Catheter (see Figure 6-71).
- The irrigation should then be attached to the bottom port on the side of the SpyScope Catheter head.
- For biopsies the guidewire must be removed from the SpyScope Catheter prior to inserting the SpyBite Biopsy Forceps.
- Biopsies are accomplished in the standard fashion (they will be small pieces).

POSTPROCEDURE

- Same as for ERCP.
- The physician should advise the patient about the resumption of anticoagulants.

SPHINCTER OF ODDI MANOMETRY

Reem Sharaiha, MD, MSc and
Mouen A. Khashab, MD

Sphincter of Oddi dysfunction (SOD) is an obstruction to the flow of bile or pancreatic juice through the sphincter of Oddi. It can occur after inflammation or due to an increased muscular contraction. Biliary and pancreatic manometry refers to the manometric measurement of sphincter of Oddi pressure. This procedure is currently considered the "gold standard" for the diagnosis of SOD. Pressure is measured directly with a triple-lumen water-perfused catheter that is passed through the duodenoscope into the bile or pancreatic duct. The proximal end of the catheter is connected to external transducers and a computerized recording device (Figure 6-74). Sphincter pressures are recorded as the catheter is slowly withdrawn from the duct and stationed within the sphincter zone. The duodenal pressure is taken from the zero reference point when measuring ductal and sphincteric pressures. A diagnosis of SOD is made based on basal sphincter of Oddi (SO) pressure elevation to ≥ 40 mm Hg in two leads and which is sustained for at least 30 seconds.

EQUIPMENT

- Triple-lumen biliary manometry catheter
- Water perfusion system (pump and transducers)
- Side-viewing endoscope (duodenoscope)
- Computer recorder
- Standard ERCP cannula of physician's choice

NURSING IMPLICATIONS

PREPROCEDURE

- Same as for ERCP.
- The patient must be free of muscle relaxants and opiates for 24 hours prior to the test (these affect sphincter pressure and alter test results).
- Patients on long-term pain medication may be difficult to sedate and may require general anesthesia.
- Remember that the manometry machine needs to be calibrated and set up prior to the procedure and this may take up to 45 minutes.

Figure 6-74. Sphincter of Oddi manometry.

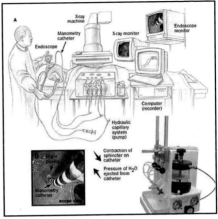

- Patients are advised to receive rectal indomethacin as a prophylactic measure against post-ERCP pancreatitis, as long as they do not have contraindication to taking nonsteroidal anti-inflammatory drugs.

INTRAPROCEDURE

- Patient positioning: Same as for ERCP.
- Patient monitoring: Same as for ERCP.
- Topical anesthetic: Same as for ERCP.
- Additional measures:
  - ▷ Same as for ERCP with sphincterotomy.
  - ▷ Since several pharmacological and hormonal agents influence sphincter of Oddi function, the endoscopist must avoid using glucagon, atropine, morphine, and other opiate analgesics and smooth muscle relaxants.
  - ▷ Propofol may be used for deep sedation.
  - ▷ Have prophylactic pancreatic stents available as they are frequently placed in this patient population due to increased risk of post-ERCP pancreatitis.

POSTPROCEDURE

- Same as for ERCP with sphincterotomy.
- Any time manipulation of the bile or pancreatic duct occurs, there is a 1% to 5% risk of causing pancreatitis (symptoms: abdominal pain, vomiting, fever, chills). There is an increased risk of post-ERCP pancreatitis is patients with suspected SOD regardless of manometry results.

- Patient positioning: Same as for ERCP.
- Patient monitoring: Same as for ERCP.
- Nursing measures that may decrease the risk of pancreatitis include the following:
  ▷ Limiting the catheter perfusion rate to 0.25 mL/lumen per minute or less.
  ▷ Use of aspiration-type manometry catheters when measuring pancreatic sphincter pressure; this type of catheter has two channels for pressure measurements and one channel to aspirate infused fluid and pancreatic juice.

ENDOSCOPIC PANCREATIC FUNCTION TESTING

Vikesh K. Singh, MD, MSc

Direct methods to assess pancreatic exocrine function have been used for decades. This was previously done using a double lumen gastroduodenal tube (Dreiling tube). The gastric lumen was used to aspirate gastric fluid and the duodenal lumen was used to aspirate pancreatic fluid. Secretin was administered to assess bicarbonate concentration as a measure of pancreatic duct cell function and cholecystokinin (CCK) was administered to assess digestive enzyme concentrations as a measure of pancreatic acinar cell function. Upper endoscopy has replaced the use of the Dreiling tube for timed collections of pancreatic fluid after IV secretagogue administration. Given the complexities of assessing pancreatic digestive enzyme concentrations after CCK administration, the secretin pancreatic function test has gained more widespread use since bicarbonate concentrations are easier to obtain using standard hospital laboratory equipment.

The patient is placed in the left lateral decubitus position. Sedation is administered. The upper endoscope is advanced into the stomach. All of the gastric fluid is aspirated. The endoscope is advanced into the descending duodenum. Secretin is intravenously injected at a concentration of 0.2 mcg/kg over 1 minute. The first 3 to 5 mL of duodenal fluid is simultaneously collected and discarded (to clear any gastric fluid from the channel) and then another 3 to 5 mL is collected into the trap. This represents the baseline or time 0 collection. Duodenal fluid is discarded and collected in a similar manner at 15, 30, 45, and 60 minutes from the time of the IV secretin administration. If the quantities of duodenal fluid output begin to fall, particularly at the later time points, the patient can be placed in a supine position to enhance pooling of fluid in the descending duodenum. All 5 specimens are sent to the laboratory on ice to assess the bicarbonate concentration. This assessment should take place no more than 6 hours after the collection of the specimens. A value of <80 mmol/L at either 30, 45, or 60 minutes is consistent with pancreatic exocrine insufficiency. An abbreviated endoscopic pancreatic function test has been validated. This involves collection of duodenal fluid at only the 30-and 45-minute time points.

EQUIPMENT

- Upper endoscope
- Secretin (0.2 mcg/kg)
- 2 to 5 suction traps
  - ▷ 2 for abbreviate endoscopic pancreatic function test (30 and 45 minute)
  - ▷ 5 for full 1 hour endoscopic pancreatic function test (0, 15, 30, 45, and 60 minutes)

NURSING IMPLICATIONS

PREPROCEDURE

- Same as standard upper endoscopy.
- Ensure that secretin is available. Sterile saline is required for suspension of secretin.
- Ask the endoscopist if full 1 hour or abbreviated pancreatic function test will be performed. Obtain and label the appropriate number of traps. Obtain a small quantity of ice.

INTRAPROCEDURE

- Same as EGD.
- Once the secretin is intravenously administered, record the time and be sure to let the endoscopist know 5 minutes before the next scheduled collection time.

POSTPROCEDURE

- Have someone from the endoscopy unit hand carry specimens to the laboratory as soon as possible.
- Same as EGD.

Chapter 6

PERITONEOSCOPY

David W. Victor III, MD and Zhiping Li, MD

Mini-laparoscopic liver biopsy refers to the peritoneoscopic examination of the liver surface and biopsy under direct visualization for the diagnosis and treatment of disorders of the liver.

EQUIPMENT

- Video monitor with video output (Figure 6-75)
- Light source (see Figure 6-75)
- Camera box (see Figure 6-75)
- CO_2 gas tank (see Figure 6-75)
- CO_2-Insufflator (see Figure 6-75) (Richard Wolf Medical Corp)
- APC unit available if needed
- Sterile peritoneoscope tray: mini fiber optic peritoneoscope (Figure 6-76a) with outer metal sheath (Figure 6-76b), Verres cannula (Figure 6-76c), high definition camera head, flexible light cable (Figure 6-76d), insufflator tubing (disposable), sterile camera drape (used if necessary, disposable)
- Prep tray: (4) sterile drapes, (4) sterile drape clamps (metal), (2) sterile prep solution (ie, Dura prep, Steri prep, or Chlora prep)
- Biopsy tray: (2) Tru-cut automated biopsy needles (disposable), 30-cc bottle of 1% lidocaine, sterile bottle of normal saline, 3-cc syringes with #23 needle, #11 scalpel blade with handle, 10-cc leur-lock syringes
- Pack of sterile 4x4 gauze

ADDITIONAL EQUIPMENT THAT MAY BE NEEDED

- 2 adhesive dressings or tape
- Bottles of formalin for biopsy specimens
- Patient identification label and pathology requisitions
- Cytology brushes
- Viral and fungal culture tubes
- Grounding pad

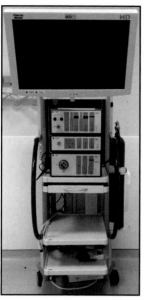

Figure 6-75. Video monitor with video output, light source, camera box, CO_2 gas tank, and CO_2-Insufflator.

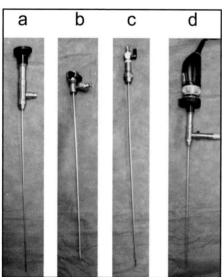

Figure 6-76. Sterile peritoneoscope tray: (a) mini fiber optic peritoneoscope (b) with outer metal sheath, (c) Verres cannula, (d) high definition camera head, flexible light cable. (Reprinted with permission from Richard Wolf Medical Corp)

Nursing Implications

Preprocedure

- Same as for upper endoscopy.
- Reassure patient about various movements in the room and the noises of the equipment.
- Prepare the room.
- All equipment listed previously should be carefully inspected and set up for procedure.
  - ▷ The CO_2 gas cylinder should be in the "on" position, and then turn on the insufflator. The insufflator must be tested to assure maximum level of gas for procedure.
  - ▷ The video system must be tested for proper functioning and patient information entered into the computer.
  - ▷ Sterile gowns, gloves, caps, shoe covers, sterile prep solution, scrub sponges, and sterile towels should be readily available for all staff involved in case needed.
  - ▷ The peritoneoscope trays should be opened on a sterile field on a rolling table.
  - ▷ A smaller sterile field should be prepared for the prep trey.
- Patient positioning: Patient should be supine with arms secured to prevent contamination of sterile field. The patient gown should be raised to expose patient from clavicle to pubis. Patient should be secured to table with patient safety straps.
- Patient monitoring: Follow sedation protocol.

Intraprocedure

- Sedation and monitoring nurse:
  - ▷ Should be at the head of the bed for monitoring the patient and administration of medications.
  - ▷ During insufflation of the peritoneal cavity the monitoring nurse may palpate the chest to check for crepitance, which would indicate passage of gas into the subcutaneous space of the chest. If crepitance is felt, notify physician for reposition of needle.
  - ▷ During insufflation the patient may feel mild discomfort or nausea while the peritoneal cavity is distending.
  - ▷ Provide medication or comfort measures as needed.

- Circulating assistant:
  - ▷ Should be within easy reach of mini-lap tower and controls for any adjustments during the case.
  - ▷ It is essential that the insufflator monitor be in direct view of the physician at all times to ensure infusion pressure stays below 20 mm Hg in the peritoneal cavity. The insufflator activates a cut-off valve when a maximum pressure limit is reached.
- Scrub nurse to assist MD with the procedure:
  - ▷ He or she should remain sterile throughout the case.
  - ▷ He or she should place the peritoneoscope cables and APC cables onto the sterile drapes and secure the cables prior to the procedure beginning.
  - ▷ He or she should attach the camera head and light source cables to the peritoneoscope.
  - ▷ After biopsy is obtained and hemostasis is achieved spontaneously or by APC, the CO_2 is allowed to escape through the trocar and the abdomen is cleaned of excess blood and sutured by physician if required. Cover with an adhesive bandage.
  - ▷ Assist the physician with taking or collecting the biopsy as requested.

POSTPROCEDURE

- The patient will be transported to the recovery area for observation for 2 hours or as indicated or ordered by physician.
- Patient should be assessed for changes in condition or vital signs.
- Abdominal puncture site should be assessed for leaking of fluid or blood, swelling, or development of hematoma.
- Patient should be assessed for severe abdominal pain, or any complaints of right shoulder pain.
- Assess patient for nausea, vomiting, abdominal distention, or fever.
- Notify the physician for any of the above or changes in condition.
- The patient may be discharged home, accompanied by an adult with discharge instructions for liver biopsy (see Appendix 2).

Peritoneoscopy

REFLUX MONITORING

Ellen Stein, MD and
Lisette Musaib-Ali, MD

Reflux is the flow of contents of the stomach upwards into the esophagus. There are several effective methods of monitoring patients for reflux including pH monitoring, wireless pH monitoring, and pH-impedance monitoring. pH monitoring involves the detection of acid. Impedance is the passage of material (gas, liquid, solid) between two measurement points on a catheter and this can be used to identify passage of material through the esophageal lumen. Reflux monitoring techniques all involve placement of a measurement device and then recording of symptoms for the duration of testing. The patient is asked to keep a diary of his or her symptoms as well as note his or her symptoms using digital trackers.

24-HOUR pH MONITORING

This test is performed to record acid reflux events in the esophagus over a 24-hour period. Twenty-four hour pH monitoring is usually performed in conjunction with esophageal motility studies, since the motility tracing can be used to determine the placement of the pH probe (5 cm above the LES)(Figure 6-77).

EQUIPMENT
- pH probe
- Surgical tape
- Water-soluble lubricant
- Digitrapper (portable data recorder from Medtronic Inc) and shoulder strap
- Buffer solutions of pH 4 and pH 7 (to calibrate the pH probe)

NURSING IMPLICATIONS

PREPROCEDURE
- The patient should have NPO for at least 8 hours.
- The patient's physician should determine whether to discontinue medications that alter pH (eg, H2 blockers, PPIs, or other medications).

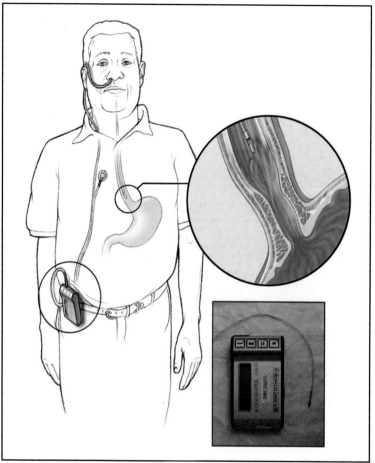

Figure 6-77. Location of ambulatory pH probe in a patient.

- A medical/surgical history, including medications, should be obtained prior to the procedure.

INTRAPROCEDURE

- The patient may sit on the side of the bed holding a glass of water with a straw for the catheter insertion.
- The first 10 cm of the catheter should be lubricated with a water-soluble lubricant. Some providers prefer a lidocaine-based lubricant, which can provide analgesia/anesthesia of the nares and the back of the throat.

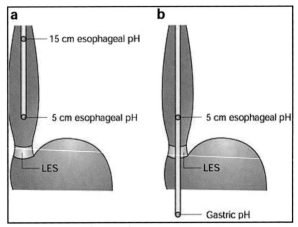

Figure 6-78. Catheter placement.

- The nurse should determine which nostril is more patent by holding each closed one at a time and asking the patient to exhale through the nose. The more patent nostril should be used.
- The nurse should begin inserting the catheter while instructing the patent to start sipping the water when he or she feels the tube in the back of his or her throat. The tube can be advanced with each swallow, allowing the peristaltic waves of the esophagus to advance the catheter to the stomach. The position can be confirmed by obtaining an acid pH (Figure 6-78).
- The tube is pulled back into the esophagus to the level of 5 cm above the LES as determined by the esophageal manometry study. Unless the patient is having constant reflux, the pH should rise to a level above 5. If unable to obtain a pH above 5, the patient should be instructed to drink water to clear the acid. The physician should be notified if this attempt fails.
- The catheter should be securely taped in place.
- Connect the pH catheter to the Digitrapper. The instrument should be turned on and placed in a shoulder strap to be worn by the patient for 24 hours.
- The patient should be informed that his or her throat might feel scratchy and sore while the tube is in place and after its removal. This is normal and should disappear a few hours after the tube is removed. The patient should have a contact number if the probe is dislodged or questions arise.

POSTPROCEDURE

- The patient should be instructed how to use the Digitrapper to record his or her meal times, medication times, changes in position (going from upright to supine, supine to upright), and gastroesophageal reflux symptoms.
- Normal daily activities may be resumed, with the exception of bathing in a tub or performing strenuous activities. Vigorous exercise could cause the patient to perspire and dislodge the electrode or probe or damage the Z-logger.
- Instruct the patient to return after 24 hours to remove the catheter. This process takes about 5 minutes. After removal, the patient may resume all normal meals, activities, and medications.

MULTICHANNEL INTRALUMINAL IMPEDANCE AND pH TESTING

Multichannel intraluminal impedance (MII) is performed to detect intraluminal bolus movement in the gut. When combined with pH testing, it allows for detection of reflux episodes in the esophagus independent of pH over a 24-hour period. Longer studies may be performed. MII-pH testing can detect the differences between acid, weakly acid, and non-acid refluxate. Twenty-four hour pH monitoring is usually performed in conjunction with esophageal motility studies as the motility tracing is used to determine the placement of the pH probe (5 cm above the LES).

EQUIPMENT

- MII-pH catheter
- Surgical tape
- Water-soluble lubricant
- ZepHr (portable data recorder from Sandhill Scientific)(Figure 6-79) and shoulder strap
- Buffer solutions of pH 4 and pH 7 (to calibrate the MII-pH catheter)

Reflux and Motility

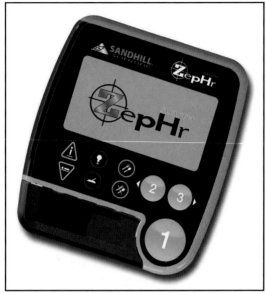

Figure 6-79. ZepHr portable data recorder.

Nursing Implications

Preprocedure

- The patient should have NPO for at least 8 hours.
- The patient's physician should determine whether to discontinue medications that alter pH (eg, H2 blockers, PPIs, or other medications).
- A medical/surgical history, including medications, should be obtained prior to the procedure.

Intraprocedure

- The patient may sit on the side of the bed holding a glass of water with a straw for the catheter insertion.
- The first 10 cm of the catheter should be lubricated with a water-soluble lubricant.
- The nurse should determine which nostril is more patent by holding each closed one at a time and asking the patient to exhale through the nose. The more patent nostril should be used.

- The nurse should begin inserting the catheter while instructing the patent to start sipping the water when he or she feels the tube in the back of his or her throat. The tube can be advanced with each swallow, allowing the peristaltic waves of the esophagus to advance the catheter to the stomach. The position can be confirmed by obtaining an acid pH (see Figure 6-78).
- The tube is pulled back into the esophagus to the level of 5 cm above the LES as determined by the esophageal manometry study. Unless the patient is having constant reflux, the pH should rise to a level above 5. If unable to obtain a pH above 5, the patient should be instructed to drink water to clear the acid. The physician should be notified if this attempt fails.
- The catheter should be securely taped in place. Usually the catheter is affixed to the side of the face with tape or a clear cellophane sticker. The catheter then can be tucked behind the ear for added protection and again affixed with tape to maintain proper position.
- Connect the pH catheter to the ZepHr. The instrument should be turned on and placed in a shoulder strap to be worn by the patient for 24 hours.
- The patient should be informed that his or her throat might feel scratchy and sore while the tube is in place and after its removal. This is normal and should disappear a few hours after the tube is removed. The patient should have a contact number if the probe is dislodged or questions arise.

POSTPROCEDURE

- The patient should be instructed on use of the ZepHr to record his or her meal times, medication times, changes in position (going from upright to supine, supine to upright), and gastroesophageal reflux symptoms.
- Normal daily activities may be resumed, with the exception of bathing in a tub or performing strenuous activities. Vigorous exercise could cause the patient to perspire and dislodge the electrode or probe or damage the Z-logger.
- Instruct the patient to return after 24 hours to remove the catheter. This process takes about 5 minutes. After removal the patient may resume all normal meals, activities, and medications.
- Patients should be instructed to keep a diary of their symptoms, medications, meals, and time periods when they are lying down for the duration of the study.

Reflux and Motility

BRAVO pH PROBE PLACEMENT

The Bravo (MedTronic Inc) probe is also used to diagnose gastroesophageal reflux disease, but it is placed during endoscopy. This is a probe that can measure pH readings from within the esophagus. Recorded pH can be sent via radio telemetry signal to a receiver worn on the patient's belt like a pager. Usually, after 24 to 48 hours of monitoring, the receiver may be returned via mail or in person and the information is downloaded by an infrared link to a computer. Longer duration studies can be performed with newer devices. The capsule should pass on its own from the body in several days. The advantages of this system are patient comfort and more normal activity level. This can be easier since the patient does not have to have a tube in the nose.

EQUIPMENT

- Bravo pH receiver
- Bravo pH capsule (Figure 6-80)
- Bravo calibration stand
- Bravo data link
- 1-AA lithium/LR6, 1.5 battery
- Calibration buffer solutions: 7.01 and 1.07
- Polygram net pH testing application software
- Sterile water, 1 500-cc bottle
- 70-90% isopropyl alcohol
- Medela vacuum pump and connecting tubing
- Same as for EGD

NURSING IMPLICATIONS

PREPROCEDURE

- Same as for EGD. Most physicians would recommend that patients cease taking PPIs for 7 days and H2 receptor antagonists for at least 2 days prior to placement of Bravo. Some physicians are interested in acid control and allow patients to continue medications. Accurately record what medications the patient has taken for 1 week prior to the procedure.
- Calibrate the Bravo capsule the day of the procedure according to the manufacturer's instructions.
- Explain diet, activity, and diary instructions to the patient before the procedure because of the sedation used.

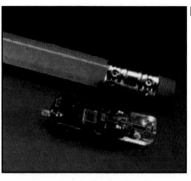

Figure 6-80. Bravo capsule.

INTRAPROCEDURE

- Same as for EGD, with the exception of the special suction set-up used in the Bravo placement. Follow manufacturer's instructions for set-up.
- A routine EGD is performed and the physician measures the centimeters from the mouth to 5 cm above the LES.
- The scope is removed.
- The Bravo capsule (on an introducer delivery device) is inserted into the mouth and down past the point in the esophagus where it will be attached. Then the device is carefully pulled back into position (see markings of measurement on the introducer). Do not lubricate the capsule prior to insertion. The lubrication will interfere with the suction capture.
- Some physicians prefer to confirm placement of the catheter under endoscopic vision, and the endoscope is reinserted into the pharynx to ensure that the capsule is within the esophageal lumen. Generous suctioning is applied after the location is confirmed. The nurse may be asked to turn off the air during this portion of the procedure.
- The nurse or technician will connect the introducer to suction and turn on the suction device when the physician signals that all is positioned well. Suction is applied to the esophageal mucosa pulling tissue into the capsule. Suction is held between 30 and 60 seconds.
- The safety (usually a white piece blocking early firing of the release button) is then removed from the introducer device by the physician or assistant.
- The physician pushes a button at the proximal end of the delivery system that fires a pin into the suctioned mucosa to hold the capsule against the esophageal wall.

- To complete release of the firing pin, while suction is still being applied, the button is gently turned to complete firing, and then nudged up into full release.
- Suction is discontinued by the nurse after deployment is completed.
- The delivery system is gently rocked off the newly placed capsule and carefully removed.

POSTPROCEDURE

- Same as for EGD, with the exception of attaching the receiver to the patient's belt before discharge and sending him or her home with written instructions and diary. The patient needs to be aware that the capsule will release in a few days time and should pass on its own. A warning should be given to the patient that MRI should be avoided until the capsule has been observed to pass, if urgent MRI is needed an x-ray can be performed to confirm its release.
- Patients should be instructed to keep a diary of their symptoms, meals, and time periods when they are lying down for the duration of the study. Medications taken before, during, and after the study must be noted.

ACID PERFUSION TEST (BERNSTEIN TEST)

The acid perfusion or Bernstein test may be used to diagnose gastroesophageal reflux disease (GERD). It is infrequently performed with the advent of the other testing modalities. It is performed in the GI laboratory by alternately infusing NS and diluted 0.1 N HCl (hydrochloric acid) into the distal esophagus. The Bernstein test confirms sensitivity to acid in the esophagus.

During the procedure, the patient is blinded to the infusion of 60 to 80 mL of 0.1 N HCl or normal saline. The infusion is introduced into a nasogastric tube (placed at 30 cm) into the esophagus at a rate of 6 to 8 mL/minute. The nurse is responsible for recording the patient's response. Reproduction of the patient's typical symptoms (on two acid infusions) may be interpreted as a positive test response. If this is the case, the physician will most likely treat the patient for GERD.

EQUIPMENT

- Two 1000-mL containers, one containing 1000 cc of normal saline, the other containing 1000 cc of 0.1 N HCl
- Y-connecting tube that attaches to each bottle and joins to form one that connects to a nasogastric tube
- 12-French nasogastric tube

- 60-cc catheter-tip syringe
- Cup of water and a straw
- Water-soluble lubricant

NURSING IMPLICATIONS

PREPROCEDURE

- The patient should have NPO after midnight prior to the test.
- The patient must be advised to allow 2 hours for the test (symptoms need to be reproduced at least twice).
- A medical/surgical history should be obtained documenting medications and allergies.
- The patient's physician should determine whether to discontinue medications that alter pH (eg, H2 blockers, PPIs, and other medications). If necessary, medications should be discontinued 2 to 7 days prior to the procedure.

INTRAPROCEDURE

- The patient should be in a sitting position with the bottles of saline and HCl located behind him or her.
- The patient is asked to swallow sips of water while the lubricated nasogastric tube is inserted through the most patent nostril. If the patient cannot tolerate the nasal tube insertion, it may be inserted through the mouth.
- Placement of the tube in the stomach is confirmed by using the stethoscope placed on the abdominal area over the stomach to listen for the "swish" of air that is forced through the tube using a 60-cc catheter-tip syringe. The tube is then withdrawn to 30 cm and taped in place.
- The nasogastric tube is connected to a Y set-up, and the saline drip is initiated. The patient must be watched carefully for symptoms, and reactions should be recorded.
- The nurse will alternate solutions without the patient's knowledge and record reactions.
- If symptoms are reproduced with HCl, the nurse should switch back to saline solution until the symptoms subside. Subsequently, symptoms must be reproduced a second time. If symptoms do not subside fully, but only lessen in severity, this must also be accurately recorded.

Reflux and Motility

POSTPROCEDURE

- The tube is removed upon completion of the study and the patient may be discharged.
- Gargling with warm salt water or using throat lozenges may relieve sore throat symptoms.
- The patient may resume a normal diet unless otherwise instructed.
- The physician may prescribe an antacid if the patient's symptoms do not abate.

BASAL ACID OUTPUT STUDY

A basal acid output (BAO) study measures the amount of acid in the stomach after fasting for 8 hours (baseline acid level). This test is performed to evaluate the effectiveness of acid suppression (with PPIs, H2 blockers, or surgical vagotomy) and to evaluate the patient for hyperacidity.

EQUIPMENT

- 12-French nasogastric tube
- Intermittent suction set-up
- 60-cc catheter-tip syringe
- Stethoscope
- Water-soluble lubricant
- Containers for collection of specimens (labeled with date, time, amount)

NURSING IMPLICATIONS

PREPROCEDURE

- The patient should have NPO after midnight prior to the test.
- A medical/surgical history, including medications, should be obtained prior to the procedure.
- The patient's physician should determine whether to discontinue medications that alter pH (eg, H2 blockers, PPIs, or other medications). If necessary, medications should be discontinued 2 to 7 days prior to the procedure.
- If the test is being done to evaluate the effectiveness of treatment, medications should be taken as prescribed until the morning of the test.

INTRAPROCEDURE

- The patient should sit on the side of the bed for insertion of the nasogastric tube.
- The first 10 cm of the tube should be lubricated. No water should be sipped, as it may alter the study results.
- Swallowing facilitates insertion of the tube.
- Placement of the tube in the stomach is confirmed by using a stethoscope to listen for the "swish" of air that is forced through the tube using a 60-cc catheter-tip syringe.
- Once placement is confirmed, stomach contents should be suctioned and placed in a labeled container (baseline specimen). Subsequent specimens should be collected at 15-minute intervals for a total of four times during the study and labeled appropriately.
- The tube should be removed after the last specimen has been obtained, and the patient may be discharged.
- Specimens should be sent to the lab for analysis. Specimens are evaluated for amount, color, consistency, pH, hydrogen ion concentration, and total acid content. This information is forwarded to the physician.

POSTPROCEDURE

- The patient may be discharged and may resume regular diet, medications, and activities.

SECRETIN STIMULATION STUDY

The secretin stimulation study is performed in the GI laboratory to detect the presence of Zollinger-Ellison syndrome (gastrinoma). This is a non-beta islet cell tumor of the pancreas, which causes large amounts of gastrin to be secreted into the blood stream. Three primary characteristics of this disease are severe peptic ulcer formation in unusual locations, gastric hypersecretion of gigantic proportions, and nonspecific islet cell tumors of the pancreas. Thickened folds of the stomach and chronic diarrhea are also prominent symptoms, but may be indicative of other diseases. Most patients with gastrinoma present with complaints of abdominal pain. During the secretin stimulation test, a baseline blood level is drawn. Then, secretin 2 cu/kg is injected intravenously. Blood samples are drawn at intervals of 2, 5, 10, 15, and 30 minutes. In patients with gastrinoma, peak serum levels occur at 2 to 5 minutes and are normal again at 15 minutes.

Reflux and Motility

EQUIPMENT

- 20-gauge or larger angiocatheter and heparin lock
- Six red-topped tubes for blood collection
- Tourniquet
- Container filled with ice (10-oz styrofoam cup)
- Vials of secretin (enough for 2 cu/kg of body weight)
- Vials of injectable saline to reconstitute secretin
- Seven 10-cc syringes (if a Vacutainer [Becton, Dickinson & Co]is used, only one 10-cc syringe is required)
- Watch or timer
- Alcohol wipes and 2x2 gauze pads with tape

NURSING IMPLICATIONS

PREPROCEDURE

- Prior to scheduling, a baseline gastrin level should be obtained.
- The patient should have NPO after midnight prior to the test.
- Discontinue PPIs and H2 blockers 72 hours prior to testing.
- Obtain a brief medical history along with allergies and medications.

INTRAPROCEDURE

- The patient may sit in a chair or lie supine depending upon his or her preference.
- An IV line is placed with a 20-gauge angiocatheter or larger and a heparin lock placed onto the angiocatheter. This facilitates access for blood drawing. There is no need to use heparin in between the blood draws; flushing with saline is sufficient to keep the line patent.
- Apply the tourniquet for each blood draw and remove it in between blood draws.
- Draw a baseline blood level, and then inject secretin 2 cu/kg slowly over 1 to 2 minutes.
- If the patient has any untoward reaction to the secretin, stop the test and call the physician immediately. Reactions to secretin are very rare, but it has been reported that a rash or hives may occur at the injection site.
- Blood samples should be drawn at intervals of 2, 5, 10, 15, and 30 minutes.

- All vials of collected blood should be kept on ice until delivery to the appropriate laboratory for analysis.

POSTPROCEDURE

- After the test is complete, the IV line should be removed and the patient may be discharged.
- The patient should be instructed to call his or her physician if the injection site becomes red or swollen.

Reflux and Motility

Esophageal Manometry Studies

Sameer Dhalla, MD, MHS and
John Clarke, MD

Conventional Manometry

Esophageal motility studies are performed to measure esophageal pressures and contractions. They may be indicated in patients having difficulty swallowing, experiencing noncardiac chest pain, and heartburn. This test measures the pressures within the esophagus by passing a long, thin, flexible manometric catheter (diameter is comparable to a nasogastric tube) into the stomach. The catheter is then pulled back slowly through the LES, through the body of the esophagus, and through the upper esophageal sphincter (UES). The transmitters placed every 5 cm on the catheter transmit the pressures to a computer. The computer prints out the information on a tracing in the form of high and low waves.

Equipment
- Manometry catheter
- Manometry machine
- Water-soluble lubricant
- 8 oz of water with a straw

Nursing Implications

Preprocedure
- The patient should have nothing to eat or drink after midnight prior to the test.
- A medical and surgical history, including medications, should be obtained before the procedure.
- The patient should discontinue use of smooth muscle relaxants or any drugs that would decrease esophageal motility for 72 hours prior to the test.
- The patient's physician should determine whether to discontinue the use of PPIs or H2 blockers at least 48 hours before the test (Figure 6-81).

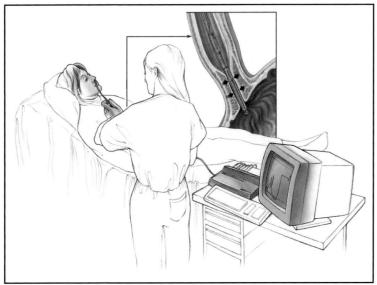

Figure 6-81. Patient set-up for esophageal motility.

INTRAPROCEDURE

- The patient may be sitting on the side of the bed holding a glass of water with a straw for the insertion of the motility catheter.
- The nurse should determine which nostril is more patent by holding each nostril closed and asking the patient to exhale though his or her nose. The more patent nostril should be used.
- The first 10 cm of the motility catheter should be lubricated with a water-soluble lubricant.
- The nurse should begin inserting the catheter, instructing the patient to start sipping water when he or she feels the tube in the back of his or her throat. The tube can be advanced with each swallow, allowing the peristaltic waves of the esophagus to advance the catheter to the stomach. If insertion is difficult, turning the patient's head to the side changes the position of the esophagus and may facilitate passage of the catheter. Do not try to force the catheter because it may cause esophageal perforation (particularly if the patient has an esophageal diverticulum).
- Once the catheter is in the stomach, the patient is instructed to lie on his or her back with the head and chest elevated (about 30 to 40 degrees).

- The catheter is attached to the computer and slowly withdrawn. This so-called "station pull-through technique" allows the boundaries of the LES to be localized.
- The patient should remain as still and quiet as possible and avoid swallowing unless instructed to do so. The test takes approximately 45 minutes to complete.

POSTPROCEDURE
- Once the tube is removed, the patient may be discharged.
- Normal meals, activities, and medications may be resumed.

HIGH-RESOLUTION MANOMETRY

Many practices and most referral centers have transitioned from the conventional manometry described previously to a system of high-resolution manometry (HRM). This technological advance provides more useful clinical information about esophageal function:

- The traditional catheter with widely-spaced transmitters is replaced by a catheter with multiple closely spaced sensors, resulting in more data points and less separation between those sites (Figure 6-82).
- Detailed color-coded topographic maps now replace the line traces of conventional manometry.
- Both the nursing staff and the patient will find HRM studies easier and more pleasant to perform:
  ▷ The pull-through technique described above is no longer required because the extra sensors outline the LES automatically.
  ▷ The HRM catheter is softer, more comfortable, and is attached to a less cumbersome apparatus (Figures 6-82 and 6-83).
  ▷ Fewer maneuvers and position changes are required, leading to a shorter overall study duration.

COMBINED MULTICHANNEL INTRALUMINAL IMPEDANCE AND MANOMENTRY

As described in "Reflux Monitoring" on p. 168, pH impedence can provide adjunct information about reflux and bolus transit through the esophagus. In certain clinical contexts where patients would benefit from both pH/impedance and manometry, the studies can be performed simultaneously using a specialized catheter with shared functionality.

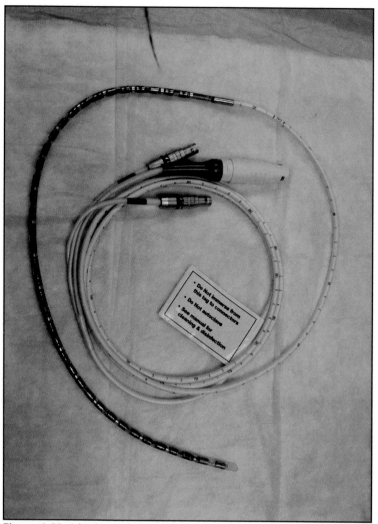

Figure 6-82. A high-resolution manometry catheter with sensors spaced only 1 cm apart. This catheter is softer and provides more information than its conventional predecessor.

Reflux and Motility

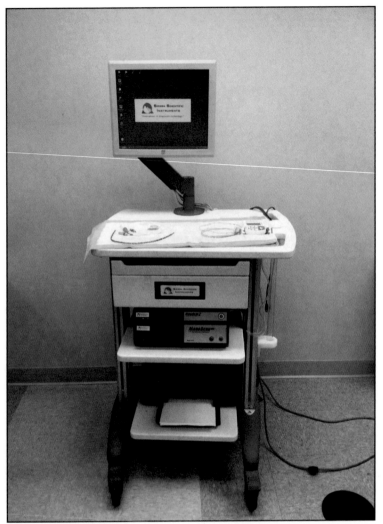

Figure 6-83. A high-resolution manometry tower.

EGD With Pneumatic Dilation for Achalasia

Ellen Stein, MD and
Rukshana Cader, MD

Achalasia is a condition of the esophagus where the LES fails to relax appropriately. The esophagus can become deformed and dilated over time due to the pressure build up within the esophagus. The classic image on barium swallow for achalasia is the bird-beak appearance of the esophagus which forms from the silhouette of the tight sphincter muscles of the LES. Most of the treatments of achalasia involve getting the muscles of the lower esophageal muscle to relax. Treatments include medical measures (botox), mechanical means to disrupt the muscle (pneumatic balloon), and different types of myotomy (peroral, laparoscopic, or open surgical incision into the muscle). In very severe cases, the esophagus itself may need to be removed to help with symptom control.

When the esophagus is treated by pneumatic dilation, the endoscopic and fluoroscopic images help guide the physician to determine when dilation or treatment is sufficient. An endoscope is used to position a guidewire. Over the guidewire, a balloon dilator can be passed into a good position to perform the pneumatic dilation. The dilating balloon will often be compressed by the force of the muscles of the LES, this compression is called the "waist." When the waist is obliterated, the balloon has been inflated to its full shape and size (like a sausage). When the waist is still present, an hourglass figure can be seen in the fluoroscopic image of the balloon. Some pneumatic balloons have markings to help the physician center the balloon so that the greatest force is applied across the LES (the area of the waist). The midpoint between the markings is where the force of dilation is strongest from the balloon and the physician will try to center the waists between these two lines.

Equipment for Achalasia Dilation

- Same as for a diagnostic EGD.
- A pediatric gastroscope may be used depending upon the tightness of the narrowing in the esophagus.
- Fluoroscopy
- Radiopaque .038-inch diameter guidewire

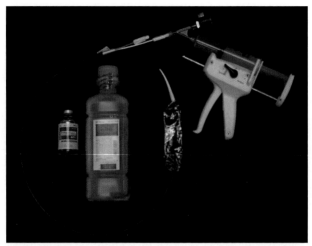

Figure 6-84. Pneumatic dilator gun attached to balloon with agents for balloon insufflation. The contrast media and saline bottle are shown here with the pneumatic balloon and dilator gun. The balloon is affixed to the gun and the syringe is preloaded with contrast prior to the dilation.

- Over-the-guidewire achalasia pneumatic balloon dilators (30 mm, 35 mm, 40 mm)
- Radiopaque half-strength contrast (50 cc distilled water plus 50 cc ionic contrast)
- Water and water-soluble lubricant for lubrication of dilator (Figure 6-84)

NURSING IMPLICATIONS

PREPROCEDURE
- Same as for a diagnostic EGD.
- Anticoagulant therapy may be adjusted or discontinued on the advice of the physician.
- Prophylactic antibiotics are not routinely needed prior to pneumatic balloon dilation.
- Patients undergoing achalasia dilation should have clear liquids for 24 to 36 hours prior to the procedure since retained food may be present in the esophagus even after a 12-hour fast.

INTRAPROCEDURE

- Same as for a diagnostic EGD.
- The patient should be positioned on the fluoroscopy table for achalasia dilations. Fluoroscopy may be necessary for guidewire placement.
- Achalasia dilation: Patient comfort and compliance are aided by bolus sedation immediately before balloon inflation (because of increased pain during dilation).
- Patient monitoring: Same as for a diagnostic EGD.
- Topical anesthetic: Same as for a diagnostic EGD.
- Additional comfort measures: Same as for a diagnostic EGD.
- Some bleeding and increased pharyngeal fluid may be expected during dilation. Frequent suctioning is imperative to prevent aspiration.

THE PROCEDURE

- Placement of the wire
  - ▷ The endoscope is inserted and the location of the LES and gastroesophageal (GE) junction should be noted. The endoscope is advanced into the stomach, and then the guidewire is advanced through the biopsy channel until it is visible in the fundus of the stomach.
  - ▷ Once the guidewire is in good position, the endoscope will be gently removed using a 1:1 technique. For each 1 cm that the endoscope is pulled back, the wire must be fed forward 1 cm to maintain position of the wire and allow for safe removal of the endoscope. The nurse may be asked to help feed the wire into position.
  - ▷ The physician may require assistance with the guidewire. The nurse should keep good control of the end of the guidewire, the guidewire itself must be in a taut, straight line to pass the balloon, but the end should be firmly grasped and coiled while the dilator is passed. A springing metal guidewire can injure bystanders if control is not maintained. The guidewire should not be allowed to slide forward or backward during insertion or removal by paying attention to the guidewire markings.
- Marking the sphincter
  - ▷ Some physicians use the position of the endoscope on fluoroscopy to note the area of planned dilation. An uncoiled paperclip can be taped to the patient's chest under fluoroscopic

guidance when it is located at the GE junction to help mark the location of the LES.

- Advancing the balloon
  - ▷ The balloon is carefully advanced over the wire. A bit of lubricant is applied to the balloon portion just before it is advanced into the esophageal lumen. While the balloon is advanced, careful attention to the wire should be paid to maintain position.
- Pneumatic balloon inflation (Figure 6-85)
  - ▷ The nurse will be asked to inflate the balloon to the appropriate pressure. Some physicians use a specific PSI by a balloon pressure inflation method, while others use a mechanical gun to inflate until the waist is lost. Inflation duration is dependent on the discretion of the physician (frequently 60 seconds).
  - ▷ Once the dilation is determined to be complete, it is important to quickly deflate the balloon. Be sure to check the method of deflation prior to starting the case. Once the balloon is deflated, notify the physician so that proper and safe removal of the balloon can be performed.

POSTPROCEDURE

- Similar to a diagnostic EGD.
- Patients should be monitored for symptoms and signs of perforation (chest pain, difficulty breathing or swallowing, or presence of subcutaneous air) following dilation. The risk of perforation is higher in achalasia dilation.
- Most patients are asked to remain NPO for sometime after the procedure to make sure no complications have occurred. Chest discomfort is common after this type of dilation.
- Many physicians routinely obtain esophagram images after pneumatic dilations, other practices only obtain esophagrams when a perforation is suspected. Good practice is to observe the patient until they are fully awake and determine the level of discomfort. After several hours of observation, if the physician is comfortable with the clinical condition of the patient, a liquid diet may be initiated.
- The patient should be able to take fluid by mouth without difficulty or pain prior to discharge.
- Diet recommendations vary, but often a soft diet is recommended for the initial recovery period.

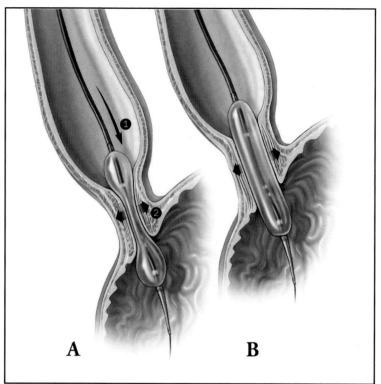

Figure 6-85. Technique of pneumatic dilation before (A) and after (B) dilation. At the start of the dilation (1) the balloon is moved into position at the GE junction, with the center of the balloon straddling the LES. At the inflation of the balloon a clear indentation can be seen within the balloon on fluoroscopy, highlighted by the contrast, (2) and this allows for the physician to note the location of the greatest balloon force directed toward the muscle layers of the LES. After complete inflation of the balloon, the indentation is lost and the dilation pressure is maintained to disrupt the LES. The dilation is completed.

Reflux and Motility

Assessing Gastrointestinal Motility

Victor Chedid, MD; Sameer Dhalla, MD, MHS; and John Clarke, MD

GI motility can be assessed by several modalities such as fluoroscopy, magnetic resonance imaging, capsule technology, or manometry. In this chapter we will discuss two of the manometric modalities: antroduodenal manometry and the wireless motility capsule (WMC). Both quantify mechanical activity of the stomach and proximal small bowel. Antroduodenal manometry provides more detailed information regarding coordination of motility and response to intervention as the catheter has multiple sensors that detect pressure changes at multiple levels, while WMC has only one sensor. On the other hand WMC is more practical since it can be done on an ambulatory basis without the insertion of any catheters and looks at whole gut motility rather than being limited to a single section of the GI tract. The choice of either modality remains at the preference of the patient and the institution.

Antroduodenal Manometry

Antroduodenal manometry is performed to measure gastric and small intestinal contractions by detecting simultaneous pressure changes at multiple levels of the gut. A long, thin, flexible manometric catheter is introduced through the nostril into the stomach and duodenum to measure these pressure changes. These changes are transmitted via the catheter to a computer and tracings in the form of waves are recorded. Antroduodenal manometry detects specific patterns in these waves that correlate with specific symptoms and GI conditions. These symptoms include abdominal pain, nausea, and vomiting associated with different clinical conditions such as gastroparesis or small bowel obstruction. These patterns help make diagnoses and direct therapeutic options.

Indications for antroduodenal manometry include unexplainable nausea and vomiting, differentiation between antral hypomotility and duodenal dysmotility, and identification of gastroduodenal motility problems in patients with delayed gastric emptying.

Equipment

- Manometry catheter* (solid-state or water-perfused catheter)
- Water-soluble lubricant
- 8 oz of water with a straw

- Medications for pharmacologic provocation of antroduodenal contractions (200 mg of erythromycin IV over 20 min, 100 mcg of octreotide SQ, or other agents based on institutional preference)
- Possible meal ingestion followed by 1 hour postprandial recording

*Types of Catheters
Two types of catheters are usually used to record antroduodenal manometry tracings.

Water-perfused Catheter:
This catheter has side holes that become occluded by sequential contraction of the gut. Water flows through the catheter at a low rate. When the holes are occluded there is resistance against the flow of water and this resistance can be measured as a change in pressure. This is then transmitted to the computer and recorded as a wave tracing. The water-perfused catheter is best suited for recordings over short periods of time, and hence is typically used to test abnormalities in the fasting states and during a meal activity only. Because hydrostatic pressure is also dependent on gravity, using a water perfused catheter requires the patient to be stationary throughout the procedure. This technology has been largely replaced by solid-state catheters but may still be used in some centers.

The following are requirements:
- Low compliance pneumohydraulic perfusion system
- Multi-lumen catheter
- External strain gauge transducer
- Degassed water in a reservoir at a constant pressure (7.5 to 15 psi by CO_2) and a constant perfusion rate (0.1 to 0.3 mL/min)

Solid-state Catheter:
This technology has widely replaced the water-perfused catheter in most centers. It is used to record intraluminal contractions from the stomach and small intestines. This catheter is more sensitive and records a higher percentage of pressure events.

The advantage of solid-state catheter is its ability to measure an ambulatory 24-hour period of contractions. The patient is usually provided with a mobile recording device attached to the solid state catheter. This allows detection of different motility patterns during different daily activities.

Reflux and Motility

Chapter 6

PREPROCEDURE

- The patient should have NPO for 8 hours prior to the procedure.
- The patient should discontinue drugs that affect motility (such as anticholinergics, metoclopramide, erythromycin, cisapride, octreotide, and narcotics) at least 48 hours prior to the procedure (unless there has been a conscious decision to measure motility on existing therapy).
- Document baseline blood pressure, pulse, respirations, oxygen saturation, level of consciousness, and pain level.
- Document drug allergies and daily medications, including dose and frequency.
- Start IV of D5/.45 NS (normal saline) or .9 normal saline if the procedure is being performed under endoscopic guidance. If the catheter is placed under fluoroscopic guidance, then this is not necessary.
- The physician should obtain an informed consent from the patient or a responsible adult.
- Obtain a medical and surgical history from the patient or responsible adult and confirm the completion of a physical exam by the physician.
- Review the discharge instructions with the patient or responsible adult.
- Ensure that a responsible adult is available to accompany the patient home if the patient is not kept in the endoscopy unit or inpatient setting for the procedure.

INTRAPROCEDURE

- The nurse should determine which nostril is more patent by holding each nostril closed and asking the patient to exhale through his or her nose. The more patent nostril should be used.
- Patient positioning depends on the way the procedure is performed.
- If performed endoscopically, use left lateral position to facilitate drainage of pharyngeal secretions. Knees should be bent toward the chest for comfort and stabilization of the patient. The patient's head may be flexed in a forward position to ease the introduction of the endoscope.
- If performed under fluoroscopic guidance, the patient may be sitting on the side of the bed holding a glass of water with a straw for the insertion of the motility catheter. The patient's head may be flexed in a forward position to ease the introduction of the endoscope.

- The first 10 cm of the motility catheter should be lubricated with a water-soluble lubricant to ease introduction.
- Catheter placement: The catheter is inserted through the nose in order to place the recording ports in the stomach and small intestines.
- If done fluoroscopically, the catheter is inserted into the nostril and the patient is instructed to take sips of water to allow the peristaltic waves of the esophagus to advance the catheter to the stomach. It is then guided through the pylorus to the small bowel under fluoroscopic guidance. In case of difficult insertion, the patient is asked to turn his or her head to the side facilitating the passage of the catheter. In case of resistance, don't use force to avoid risk of perforation or trauma. Verification of the placement of the recording ports in the proper position is done fluoroscopically.
- If done using upper endoscopy, which is the modality used at our institution, the motility catheter is guided into the small bowel by the endoscope. Due to the sensitivity of the recording sensor, this is most safely performed by grasping a string tied to the distal tip of the catheter and using that to advance the motility catheter to the small bowel (similar to the endoscopic insertion of a nasoduodenal [ND] tube).
- During the first 3 hours of the recording, fasting motility is recorded. After that, a provocation of the gut is done either pharmacologically or by giving the patient a meal and a recording of the gut activity is made.
- Patient monitoring: Document EKG, blood pressure, respiratory rate, and pulse oximetry every 15 minutes during the procedure or more often if the patient's condition warrants in case the procedure is done endoscopically.
- Pain level must be monitored during the procedure.
- Emergency equipment including suction, oxygen, and crash cart must be readily available.
- Topical anesthetic (viscous lidocaine swish and swallow or 4% lidocaine spray) may be used.
- Additional comfort measures such as soothing, calming words of encouragement along with light back massage may improve the patient's comfort.

Reflux and Motility

POSTPROCEDURE

- Monitor vital signs, blood pressure, pulse, oxygen saturation, level of consciousness, and pain level until they have returned to baseline.
- The patient may be discharged home, accompanied by an adult with discharge instructions.
- Different protocols exist for postprandial and post medication monitoring and this can be performed as an outpatient or inpatient based on institution preference.
- The physician should be notified if the patient experiences vomiting, abdominal pain, distension, or fever.

WIRELESS MOTILITY CAPSULE USING A pH/ PRESSURE-SENSING CAPSULE (SMARTPILL)

The WMC is a wireless device used to evaluate whole gut and regional gut transit and motility. By measuring luminal pH, pressure, and temperature, it helps determine gastric emptying time, small bowel transit time, colonic transit time, and whole gut transit time without a need for radiation exposure and on an outpatient basis. This technique is FDA approved for evaluation of gastric emptying in patients with suspected gastroparesis, and for the evaluation of colonic and whole gut motility in patients with chronic constipation who are suspected to have slow transit. Common indications include nausea, vomiting, bloating, heartburn, constipation, and early satiety.

EQUIPMENT

- Visualizing pH and pressure capsule (indigestible capsule with a temperature, pressure, and pH sensors)* (Figure 6-86)
- Standardized nutrient bar (SmartBar)
- 50 cc of water
- Data receiver (Figure 6-87)
- Personal computer
- Software for analyzing images (SmartPill MotiliGI Software)

*The capsule functions for 120 to 144 hours after activation and samples data at regular intervals once every 20 seconds in the first 24 hours and then once every 40 sec. Thereafter the information is transmitted to the data receiver, which will be analyzed and read using specific software (Figure 6-88).

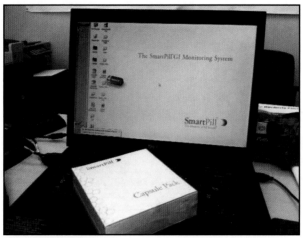

Figure 6-86. SmartPill.

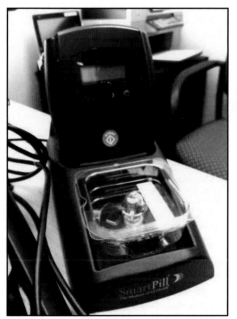

Figure 6-87. Data receiver and docking station.

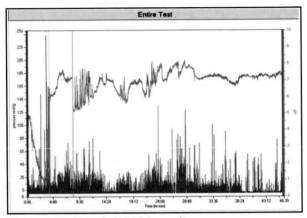

Figure 6-88. Sample WMC Recording.

PREPROCEDURE

- Instruct the patient to fast overnight.
- Charge the battery pack the evening before the procedure according to the manufacturer's instruction.
- On the morning of the procedure, calibrate the receiver and download the needed information as per the manufacturer's instructions.
- The patient is instructed not to smoke prior to and during the test.
- Iron and sucralfate are withheld several days prior to the test.
- Motility medications (metoclopramide, anticholinergics, erythromycin, cisapride, octreotide, and narcotics) are to be withheld for 48 hours after taking the WMC; unless there has been a conscious decision to evaluate motility on the patient's current regimen.
- Any medications that affect acidity are to be stopped according to the following: PPIs are to be stopped 7 days prior to the test, H2 blockers are to be stopped for 48 hours, and antacids for 24 hours after taking the pill. (This is necessary as the regional transit is determined largely based on pH changes that may be altered by these medications.)
- Obtain a brief medical and surgical history.
- Ask the patient for presence of implanted electronic devices (pacemakers or defibrillators), pregnancy, Zenker's diverticulum, fistulae or stricture, swallowing disorders, history of GI surgery in past 3 months, Crohn's disease, and diverticulosis all of which are at least relative contraindications.

- The test is contraindicated in cases of potential small bowel obstruction.
- Make sure the patient has no MRIs scheduled in the 2 weeks following the test.
- The physician should obtain an informed consent from the patient or responsible adult, given the potential risk of capsule retention/obstruction.

PROCEDURE

- The patient is instructed to consume the nutrient bar, followed by the WMC with 50 cc of water.
- The data receiver is held in place by a belt or suspender, and must be kept within 3 feet of the patient at all times.

POSTPROCEDURE

- The patient must have nothing to eat except sips of water (up to 1 cup total) for the next 6 hours and then can resume a normal diet.
- Some protocols instruct the patient to ingest a meal or occasionally Ensure (Abbott Laboratories) at 6 hours to assess postprandial response.
- The patient is instructed to push the event button and to keep a diary of symptoms with specific timing.
- The patient is discharged home and can perform normal daily activity.
- The patient is instructed to refrain from alcohol and vigorous exercise until after the WMC has passed.
- The receiver has a signal indicator: The "radar symbol" signifies the capsule is received and documenting, an "X" means the capsule is out of range or has exited the body. The receiver should be kept no further than 3 feet from the patient.
- Once the WMC has been evacuated from the body, the data receiver should detect an abrupt drop in pH and should indicate an "X."
- The patient is instructed to return the receiver to the physician's office or to mail it back (provide the patient with proper mailing boxes) after completion of the data recording.
- If the capsule does not pass in 5 days, the patient should notify his or her physician so an abdominal x-ray can be performed to document position of the WMC and ensure WMC removal. At our institution, this is typically arranged 2 weeks post-test completion if the WMC is not documented to have left the body.

Reflux and Motility

Chapter 6

ANORECTAL MANOMETRY

Victor Chedid, MD; Sameer Dhalla, MD, MHS; and John Clarke, MD

Anorectal manometry (ARM) is the most commonly performed test of anorectal function and physiology. It helps assess anorectal sphincter function, mechanisms of defecation and continence, rectal sensation, rectal compliance, and anorectal reflexes. Anorectal disorders affect 20% of the population, and ARM helps delineate the underlying cause and directs optimal management. With the proper history and clinical assessment, ARM helps confirm clinical diagnoses and provides additional information that cannot be elicited clinically. One prospective study showed ARM to be useful in 88% of patients with symptoms suggestive of defecatory dysfunction and that has been the experience as well at our institution.

INDICATIONS
- Refractory/chronic constipation
- Fecal and/or flatulence incontinence
- Preoperative evaluation for anorectal surgery (anal fissure, anal fistula, anorectal cancer, reversal of ileostomy/colostomy)
- Postoperative evaluation for reversal of colostomy
- Behavioral modification conditioning (biofeedback) technique to improve bowel control in patients with incontinence or dyssynergia
- Suspected cases of scleroderma, dermatomyositis, Hirschsprung's disease

CONTRAINDICATIONS
- Severe or unstable medical or psychological disorders
- Infectious diarrhea
- Anal or rectal disease

EQUIPMENT
The ARM consists of four main components:
1. Anorectal manometry catheter/probe (pressure-sensing device): There are two different types of probes used to measure intraluminal pressures:

▷ Solid-state microtransducer: Thin, flexible tube with micro-transducers that directly sense pressure. It provides an accurate recording but is more expensive and fragile.

▷ Water-perfused/sleeve catheter or water/air-filled balloon catheter: Thin, plastic tube with 4 to 8 side holes and a central channel for balloon inflation that relies on the pneumohydraulic pump to measure pressures. It is simple and cheaper, but is more difficult to calibrate and cannot be used in the sitting position to perform studies.

In addition, both probes can be arranged with multiple sensors which are spaced more closely than typical to provide a high-resolution topographic profile of the anorectal region. This provides more detailed information; however, the clinical gain from this technology as opposed to standard sensor/channel spacing is still under investigation. Recently, high-definition solid-state catheters have also been developed that provide three dimensional representation of the sphincter and may provide more accurate localization of focal contractions and defects. The potential clinical uses of this high-definition probe are still being investigated.

2. Amplifier/recorder which converts signals to digital data
3. Monitor for displaying the recordings
4. Software for data analysis

OTHER EQUIPMENT NEEDED

- Catheter sheath (optional for solid-state systems only)
- 4x4 sponges
- Talc powder
- 60-cc leur-lock syringe
- Stopcock
- Water-soluble lubricant
- Balloon to affix to catheter

PATIENT PREPARATION

Technically, there is no bowel preparation or dietary restrictions for this study. At our institution, we request that the patient take two enemas on the morning of the study to empty their rectum; however, this is optional. We do not stop routine medications before the study.

Chapter 6

Procedure

- Explain the procedure to the patient (purpose of the study, sensations to expect during the study, and all the maneuvers to be performed according to indication)
- Position the patient on his or her left lateral side, with his or her hips and knees flexed at 90 degrees.
- Perform a digital rectal exam (DRE):
  ▷ Inspect the anus and surrounding area for fissures, scars, hemorrhoids.
  ▷ Check for stool in the vault.
  ▷ Assess resting and squeeze sphincter tone and assess for potential defects by asking the patient to bear down.
  ▷ Note any anatomical abnormalities that prevent proper insertion of the catheter.
- Lubricate the probe with the water-based lubricant.
- Insert the lubricated probe into the rectum at approximately 10 cm from the tip of the balloon. Make sure the sphincter pressure band is in the center of the lower section on the display.
- Immobilize the probe and allow the patient 3 to 4 minutes to become accustomed to the probe.
- Encourage the patient to relax and breathe normally.
- Adjust the proximal and distal pressure boundaries of the anal sphincter using the appropriate software.
- Begin recording using the appropriate motility software.

Assessment of Resting Anal Sphincter Pressure

This is to assess the baseline sphincter pressure, which reflects, primarily internal anal sphincter pressure (IAS). The preferred technique is the stationary technique, which takes the highest pressure at any level in the anal canal as the maximum resting sphincter pressure. The normal pressure is usually between 50 to 80 mm Hg. These normative data vary based on the catheter and motility equipment utilized and it is best to check with the specific motility catheter manufacturer used to obtain their normative data.

Assessment of Squeeze Anal Sphincter Pressure

This primarily assesses the strength of the external anal sphincter (EAS) during a voluntary squeeze. Ask the patient to squeeze the anus for as long as possible (preferably at least 20 seconds), and then repeat this after 1 minute of rest. The highest sphincter pressure recorded at any level of the anal canal is considered the maximum anal squeeze pressure. A weak squeeze may be secondary to either a neurogenic or myogenic dysfunction, sphincter injury, or other less common abnormality.

ABDOMINO-PELVIC REFLEX (COUGH REFLEX TEST)

This test determines the integrity of the anal sphincter continence during an abrupt increase of intra-abdominal pressure. Ask the patient to cough, or blow a balloon, twice with a 1-minute resting interval.

ATTEMPTED DEFECATION

Ask the patient to strain and to bear down as if to defecate while lying on the bed, and repeat after 30 seconds of rest. This test measures the pressure changes in the rectum and anal sphincter during attempted defecation and the coordination with abdominal muscle contraction. Normally, rectal pressure should increase and anal sphincter pressure should decrease. Dyssenergic defecation is the inability to perform this coordinated maneuver leading to functional obstruction of stool passage.

There are four types of dyssenergic defecation:

1. Type 1: The patient generates an adequate pushing force (increase in intrarectal pressure) with a paradoxical increase in anal sphincter pressure.
2. Type 2: The patient is unable to generate an adequate pushing force, with a paradoxical increase in anal sphincter pressure.
3. Type 3: The patient can produce an adequate pushing force with either absent or incomplete sphincter relaxation.
4. Type 4: The patient cannot produce an adequate pushing force with no anal sphincter relaxation.

RECTOANAL INHIBITORY REFLEX

Distention of the rectal wall induces relaxation of the IAS mediated by the myenteric plexus in a phenomenon known as the rectoanal inhibitory reflex (RAIR). This reflex is elicited by inflating the intrarectal balloon. To perform this maneuver, rapidly inflate the balloon with 20 cc of air then withdraw the air rapidly. Repeat incrementally with 40 cc, 60 cc, or until a sustained relaxation is produced. The lowest balloon volume that induces anal sphincter relaxation and causes sustained relaxation is recorded. The absence of RAIR is typical in Hirschsprung's disease (rare in adults).

Reflux and Motility

Sensorimotor Response (Sensation Test)

The sensorimotor response is produced when the rectum is distended, resulting in a contractile motor response from the anal sphincter/puborectalis region. This results in the desire to defecate. Abnormal rectal sensation plays a role in the pathophysiology of many colorectal problems such as chronic constipation. Some of these problems can be reversed by behavioral modification conditioning or biofeedback training.

- Confirm that the balloon is free of air.
- Slowly fill the balloon with air to 10 cc. After 20 seconds, deflate the balloon fully and wait 20 seconds. Then inflate the balloon in 10-cc increments and deflate each time with 20 seconds in between each inflation until the patient feels the sensation of the balloon. At that point, mark the volume required to achieve initial sensation.
- Next, continue filling the balloon, now at 20-cc increments until the patient feels the urge to defecate. At that point, mark the volume required to achieve "urge."
- Continue filling the balloon until the patient feels discomfort. Note that the balloon should be inflated to a maximum volume of 200 cc for adults or 100 cc for pediatric patients or until the maximum tolerable volume is reached.
- Deflate the balloon and ensure that all air is removed.

Discontinuation of the Probe

After completion of all indicated maneuvers, end software recording and gently remove the probe from the patient. Provide him or her with a washcloth and privacy to change.

Standard Report of Anorectal Manometry

- General information
- Patient demographics
- Procedure details: Indication(s) for test, orientation, number and location of sensors, balloon location and length, documentation of calibration
- Anal sphincter pressures: Resting sphincter pressure (mm Hg), squeeze sphincter pressure (mm Hg), duration of sustained squeeze (seconds), cough reflex (rectal and anal pressure [mm Hg]), attempted defecation (rectal and anal pressure [mm Hg]), RAIR (absent or present, minimal volume that elicits the reflex)

- Rectal sensation: Threshold for first sensation (mL), desire to defecate (mL), urgency (mL), maximum tolerable volume (mL)
- Comments/ interpretation/summary: Summarizing the findings
- Diagnosis
- Identifier/signature

COMPLICATIONS OF ANORECTAL MANOMETRY

This procedure is usually a very safe one and complications are rare. There have been rare reports of serious complications such as colon perforation. To prevent such problems, the probe should be inserted and removed gently, the intraluminal pressure should be monitored during balloon distention, and the balloon must be deflated promptly if the patient complains of pain.

Reflux and Motility

Botulinum Toxin Injection in the Upper Gastrointestinal Tract
Stuart K. Amateau, MD, PhD

Botulinum toxin (Botox) is a potent neuromuscular blocker. It is used in the upper GI tract to relax smooth muscle. In the last decade its use has expanded to include smooth muscle disorders such as achalasia, diffuse esophageal spasm, dysphagia from nonspecific esophageal motility disorders, isolated hypertension of the LES, sphincter of Oddi dysfunction, oropharyngeal dysphagia, and gastroparesis. More recently, physicians have injected botulinum toxin into the muscle layer of the gastric antrum to inhibit peristalsis and achieve modest gastroparesis as a method of early satiety and weight loss.

EQUIPMENT
- Same as for a diagnostic EGD.
- Sclerotherapy needle
- Vial of botulinum toxin (100 units); upwards of 500 units in antral injections for weight loss
- 10-cc syringe for botulinum toxin and 3-cc syringe for saline to flush the residual toxin from the sclerotherapy needle

NURSING IMPLICATIONS

PREPROCEDURE
- Same as for a diagnostic EGD.
- Procedure for preparation of botulinum toxin:
  - ▷ Keep vial frozen until ready to use.
  - ▷ Check with the physician as to the concentration of botulinum toxin and add appropriate volume of normal saline to the vial for reconstitution, taking care not to cause bubbles, as air denatures the toxin.
  - ▷ Do not agitate the vial violently, as this causes denaturization of the mixture.
  - ▷ Draw up the botulinum toxin solution into a 10-cc syringe.
  - ▷ Flush the solution through a standard sclerotherapy needle; this uses about 1 to 2 cc of the solution.
  - ▷ The physician will then direct the nurse to inject incremental doses into the targeted area (Figure 6-89).

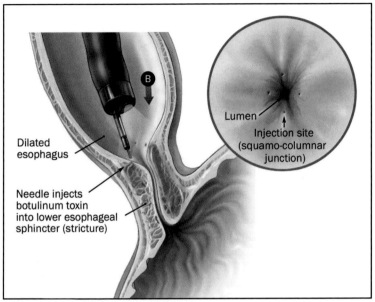

Figure 6-89. Endoscopic technique of botulinum toxin injection into the LES.

INTRAPROCEDURE

- Patient positioning: Same as for a diagnostic EGD.
- Patient monitoring: Same as for a diagnostic EGD.
- Topical anesthetic: Same as for a diagnostic EGD.
- It is necessary to use a 3-cc syringe filled with saline to flush the remaining toxin.
- Additional comfort measures: Same as for a diagnostic EGD.
- There are no special disposal instructions when using botulinum toxin.
- Needle and glass vial disposal should be performed in the usual manner in accordance with hospital waste policy.

POSTPROCEDURE

- Same as for a diagnostic EGD.
- Systemic complications are rare but include transient skin rash.
- Local side effects may be related to the targeted sphincter or organ (eg, esophageal reflux as a result of lowering esophageal pressure).

Reflux and Motility

Chapter 6

ANTIBIOTIC PROPHYLAXIS FOR GI ENDOSCOPY

Rosa Maria Fusco, RN, BSN, CGRN

Clinically significant infections after endoscopy are extremely rare. The purpose of antibiotic prophylaxis is to reduce the risk of infectious complications. Antibiotic prophylaxis is dependent upon the procedure to be performed, associated endoscopic findings, and patient-specific risk factors. The American Society for Gastrointestinal Endoscopy (ASGE) developed guidelines for appropriate use of antibiotics during GI endoscopy in common clinical situations. Guidelines are based on review of the medical literature and recommendations of expert consultants. Therefore, the guidelines are not a rule but to advise a course of treatment for specific procedural interventions. These guidelines may be revised as necessary to account for changes in technology, new data, or other aspects of clinical practice. Due to insufficient data, it is no longer recommended to administer prophylactic antibiotics to safeguard against infective endocarditis.

When a PEG placement is performed, the patient should receive prophylactic antibiotics 1 hour prior to the procedure. It is also suggested that patients be covered with antibiotics for drainage of a cystic lesion in the GI tract. Antibiotics such as cefoxitin and cefotetan have been more commonly used in recent years instead of ampicillin and gentamicin. Antibiotic prophylaxis for GI endoscopic procedures is described in Table 6-2.

General GI

TABLE 6-2. ANTIBIOTIC PROPHYLAXIS FOR GASTROINTESTINAL ENDOSCOPIC PROCEDURES

MEDICAL CONDITION	PROCEDURE	PROPHYLAXIS
All cardiac conditions	Any endoscopic procedure	No
All patients	PEG placement	Yes
Bile duct obstruction in the absence of cholangitis	ERCP with complete drainage	No
Bile duct obstruction in the absence of cholangitis	ERCP with incomplete drainage (PSC, hilar strictures)	Yes; continue antibiotics after the procedure
Cirrhosis with acute GI bleeding	Required for all patients regardless of endoscopic procedures	Upon admission
Cystic lesions along GI tract (including mediastinum)	EUS-FNA	Yes
Prosthetic joints	Any endoscopic procedure	No
Prosthetic valve	Any endoscopic procedure	No
Solid lesion along upper GI tract	EUS-FNA	No
Solid lesion along lower GI tract	EUS-FNA	Insufficient data to make recommendation
Sterile pancreatic fluid collection	ERCP	Yes

Chapter 6

MANAGEMENT OF PATIENTS ON ANTICOAGULATION THERAPY

Libbie L. Monroe, RN, BSN, CGRN and Toshunia F. Robinson, RN, BSN

The ASGE has developed guidelines for the management of patients that are on anticoagulation therapy prior to endoscopic procedures. These guidelines should be used as a tool for a gastroenterologist to manage patients that are scheduled to undergo an endoscopic procedure.

Coagulopathy is a pathologic condition that can affect the ability of the blood to clot. This condition can cause prolonged or excessive bleeding, which may occur spontaneously or following a medical procedure such as an endoscopy.

Special considerations during endoscopy include the following:

PREPROCEDURE

- Verify patient's current prothrombin time (PT), partial thromboplastin time (PTT), platelet level, and international normalized ratio (INR) if biopsy, dilation, or therapeutic procedures are contemplated.
- If PT, PTT, platelet level, or INR are not within normal limits, the physician may order fresh frozen plasma (FFP) or platelets. In addition, the physician may consider postponing the procedure to allow time for corrective actions.
- Endoscopy procedures have been divided into two groups: low-risk procedures and high-risk procedures (Table 6-3).
- Low-risk procedures generally do not require any change in management of the patient's anticoagulation/antiplatelet therapy. It is important to note that patients requiring homeostasis should be considered at high risk because of the possibility of rebleeding.
- Patient's medical conditions are also separated into low-risk and high-risk categories. Patients that fall into the high-risk category should have a multidisciplinary consultation between cardiology, hematology, and gastroenterology prior to having an endoscopy procedure (Table 6-4).
- To help prevent thromboembolic events from occurring antithrombotic agents are used to treat patients with certain cardiovascular conditions (Table 6-5).
- The gastroenterologist must consider factors such as urgency of procedure, risk of bleeding due to antithrombotic therapy, risk of

TABLE 6-3. PROCEDURE RISK FOR BLEEDING

LOW-RISK PROCEDURE	HIGH-RISK PROCEDURE
Diagnostic (EGD, colonoscopy, flexible sigmoidoscopy) including biopsy	Polypectomy
ERCP without sphincterotomy	Biliary or pancreatic sphincterotomy
EUS without FNA	Pneumatic or balloon dilation in achalasia
Enteroscopy and diagnostic balloon-assisted enteroscopy	PEG placement
Capsule endoscopy	Therapeutic balloon-assisted enteroscopy
Enteral stent deployment without dilation	EUS with FNA Endoscopic hemostasis Tumor ablation by any technique Cystogastrostomy Varices treatment Endoscopic mucosal resection Esophageal stenting Thermal ablation and coagulation

Reprinted with permission from ASGE Standards of Practice Committee; Anderson MA, Ben-Menachem T, Gan SI, et al. Management of antithrombotic agents for endoscopic procedures. *Gastrointest Endosc.* 2009;70(6): 1060-1070. doi: 10.1016/j.gie.2009.09.040.

General GI

bleeding due to interventions during the endoscopy, and risk of complication due to interruption in their antithrombotic therapy.

INTRAPROCEDURE

Have equipment for hemostatis readily available. Anticipation of bleeding episodes and swiftness of action is paramount to a positive outcome. (see "EGD for Hemostasis in Patients With Upper Gastrointestinal Bleeding" on p. 41).

TABLE 6-4. CONDITION RISK FOR THROMBOEMBOLIC EVENT	
LOW-RISK CONDITION	HIGH-RISK CONDITION
Uncomplicated or paroxysmal nonvalvular atrial fibrillation	Atrial fibrillation associated with valvular heart disease, prosthetic valves, active congestive heart failure, left ventricular ejection fraction <35%, a history of a thromboembolic event, hypertension, diabetes mellitus, or age >75 years
Bioprosthetic valve	Mechanical valve in the mitral position
Mechanical valve in the aortic position	Mechanical valve in any position and previous thromboembolic event
Deep vein thrombosis	Recently (<1 years) placed coronary stent Acute coronary syndrome Nonstented percutaneous coronary intervention after myocardial infarction
Reprinted with permission from ASGE Standards of Practice Committee; Anderson MA, Ben-Menachem T, Gan SI, et al. Management of antithrombotic agents for endoscopic procedures. *Gastrointest Endosc.* 2009;70(6): 1060-1070. doi: 10.1016/j.gie.2009.09.040.	

POSTPROCEDURE

- Monitor for signs of bleeding:
    - ▷ Significant decrease in blood pressure
    - ▷ Increased heart rate
    - ▷ Changes in mental status
    - ▷ Vomiting blood
    - ▷ Blood in stool
    - ▷ Weakness
    - ▷ Dizziness or faintness
    - ▷ Shortness of breath
    - ▷ Crampy abdominal pain
    - ▷ Pallor

Table 6-5. Antithrombotic Drugs: Duration of Action and Routes for Reversal

DRUG CLASS	SPECIFIC AGENT(S)	DURATION OF ACTION	ELECTIVE	ROUTES OF REVERSAL
Antiplatelet agent	Aspirin	10 days	NA	Transfuse platelets
	NSAIDs	Varies	NA	Transfuse platelets
	Dipyridamole	2 to 3 days	Hold	Transfuse platelets
	Thienopyridines (clopi-drogrel, Ticlopidine)	3 to 7 days	Hold	Transfuse platelets
	GP IIb/IIIa inhibitors(tirofiban, abciximab, eptifibatide)	Varies	NA	Transfuse platelets; in case of overdose agents can be removed with dialysis
Anticoagulants	Warfarin	3 to 5 days	Hold	FFP ± vitamin K, consider protamine sulfate*
	Unfractionated Heparin	4 to 6 hours	Hold	Hold or consider protamine sulfate*
	LMWH	12 to 24 hours	Hold	Hold or consider protamine sulfate*

NA, Not applicable; NSAID, nonsteroidal anti-inflammatory drug; GP, glycoprotein; FFP, fresh frozen plasma; LMWH, low molecular weight heparin. *Caution: Can cause severe hypotension and anaphylaxis

Reprinted with permission from ASGE Standards of Practice Committee; Anderson MA, Ben-Menachem T, Gan SI, et al. Management of antithrombotic agents for endoscopic procedures. *Gastrointest Endosc.* 2009;70(6): 1060-1070. doi: 10.1016/j.gie.2009.09.040.

TABLE 6-6. TIMING OF REINSTITUTION OF ANTICOAGULANT/ANTIPLATELET THERAPY AFTER GASTROINTESTINAL ENDOSCOPY

DRUG	TIMING OF REINSTITUTION	SPECIAL CONSIDERATIONS
Aspirin/ NSAIDs	Next day	
Warfarin	Same night	Consider recommencing > 3 days in case of therapeutic procedure
Heparin	2 to 6 hrs after procedure	
LMWH	24 hrs after procedure	Higher risk procedure 48 to 72 hrs after and lower dose
Clopidogrel	Next day	Consider delayed reinstitution if higher risk procedure performed

Reprinted by permission from Macmillan Publishers Ltd: The American Journal of Gastroenterology, Kwok A, Faigel DO. Management of anticoagulation before and after gastrointestinal endoscopy. *Am J Gastroenterol.* 2009;104(12):3085-3097; quiz 3098, copyright 2009

The reinstitution of anticoagulant/antiplatelet therapy after endoscopy procedures must be diligent to avoid an untoward event. The basic recommendation for the reinstitution of anticoagulant/antiplatelet therapy after a GI procedure can be found in Table 6-6.

Generally, low-risk procedures do not require any changes in anticoagulant or antiplatelet therapy. However, high-risk procedures are less clear-cut, which requires the balance of perceived thromboembolic and bleeding risks. Patients should be informed of signs and symptoms of the occurrence of bleeding, and instructed to promptly seek medical care when needed.

ACID PERFUSION TEST (BERNSTEIN TEST)

Mouen A. Khashab, MD

The acid perfusion or Bernstein test may be used to diagnose gastroesophageal reflux disease (GERD). It is performed in the GI laboratory by alternately infusing normal saline and diluted 0.1 N HCl (hydrochloric acid) into the distal esophagus. The Bernstein test confirms sensitivity to acid in the esophagus.

During the procedure, the patient is blinded to the infusion of 60 to 80 mL of 0.1 N HCl or normal saline. The infusion is introduced into a nasogastric tube (placed at 30 cm) into the esophagus at a rate of 6 to 8 mL/minute. The nurse is responsible for recording the patient's response. Reproduction of the patient's typical symptoms (on two acid infusions) may be interpreted as a positive test response. If this is the case, the physician will most likely treat the patient for GERD.

EQUIPMENT

- Two 1000-mL containers, one containing 1000 cc of normal saline, the other containing 1000 cc of 0.1 N HCl
- Y-connecting tube that attaches to each bottle and joins to form one that connects to a nasogastric tube
- 12-French nasogastric tube
- 60-cc catheter-tip syringe
- Cup of water and a straw
- Water-soluble lubricant
- Nursing Implications

PREPROCEDURE

- The patient should have NPO after midnight prior to the test.
- The patient must be advised to allow 2 hours for the test (symptoms need to be reproduced at least twice).
- A medical/surgical history should be obtained, documenting medications and allergies.
- The patient's physician should determine whether to discontinue medications that alter pH (eg, H2 blockers, PPIs, and other medications). If necessary, medications should be discontinued 2 to 7 days prior to the procedure.

General GI

INTRAPROCEDURE

- The patient should be in a sitting position with the bottles of saline and HCl located behind him or her.
- The patient is asked to swallow sips of water while the lubricated nasogastric tube is inserted through the most patent nostril. If the patient cannot tolerate the nasal tube insertion, it may be inserted through the mouth.
- Placement of the tube in the stomach is confirmed by using the stethoscope placed on the abdominal area over the stomach to listen for the "swish" of air that is forced through the tube using a 60-cc catheter-tip syringe. The tube is then withdrawn to 30 cm and taped in place.
- The nasogastric tube is connected to a Y set-up, and the saline drip is initiated. The patient must be watched carefully for symptoms, and reactions should be recorded.
- The nurse will alternate solutions without the patient's knowledge and record reactions.
- If symptoms are reproduced with HCl, the nurse should switch back to saline solution until the symptoms subside. Subsequently, symptoms must be reproduced a second time. If symptoms do not subside fully, but only lessen in severity, this must also be accurately recorded.

POSTPROCEDURE

- The tube is removed upon completion of the study and the patient may be discharged.
- Gargling with warm salt water or using throat lozenges may relieve sore throat symptoms.
- The patient may resume a normal diet unless otherwise instructed.
- The physician may prescribe an antacid if the patient's symptoms do not abate.

General GI

BASAL ACID OUTPUT TEST
Mouen A. Khashab, MD

A basal acid output (BAO) study measures the amount of acid in the stomach after fasting for 8 hours (baseline acid level). This test is performed to evaluate the effectiveness of acid suppression (with PPIs, H2 blockers, or surgical vagotomy) and to evaluate the patient for hyperacidity.

EQUIPMENT
- 12-French nasogastric tube
- Intermittent suction set-up
- 60-cc catheter-tip syringe
- Stethoscope
- Water-soluble lubricant
- Containers for collection of specimens (labeled with date, time, and amount)

NURSING IMPLICATIONS

PREPROCEDURE
- The patient should have NPO after midnight prior to the test.
- A medical/surgical history, including medications, should be obtained prior to the procedure.
- The patient's physician should determine whether to discontinue medications that alter pH (eg, H2 blockers, PPIs, or other medications). If necessary, medications should be discontinued 2 to 7 days prior to the procedure.
- If the test is being done to evaluate the effectiveness of treatment, medications should be taken as prescribed until the morning of the test.

INTRAPROCEDURE
- The patient should sit on the side of the bed for insertion of the nasogastric tube.
- The first 10 cm of the tube should be lubricated. No water should be sipped, as it may alter the study results.
- Swallowing facilitates insertion of the tube.

General GI

- Placement of the tube in the stomach is confirmed by using a stethoscope to listen for the "swish" of air that is forced through the tube using a 60-cc catheter-tip syringe.
- Once placement is confirmed, stomach contents should be suctioned and placed in a labeled container (baseline specimen). Subsequent specimens should be collected at 15-minute intervals for a total of four times during the study and labeled appropriately.
- The tube should be removed after the last specimen has been obtained, and the patient may be discharged.
- Specimens should be sent to the lab for analysis. Specimens are evaluated for amount, color, consistency, pH, hydrogen ion concentration, and total acid content. This information is forwarded to the physician.

POSTPROCEDURE

- The patient may be discharged and may resume regular diet, medications, and activities.

SECRETIN STIMULATION STUDY

Mouen A. Khashab, MD

The secretin stimulation study is performed in the GI laboratory to detect the presence of Zollinger-Ellison syndrome (gastrinoma). This is a nonbeta islet cell tumor of the pancreas, which causes large amounts of gastrin to be secreted into the blood stream. Three primary characteristics of this disease are severe peptic ulcer formation in unusual locations, gastric hypersecretion of gigantic proportions, and nonspecific islet cell tumors of the pancreas. Thickened folds of the stomach and chronic diarrhea are also prominent symptoms, but may be indicative of other diseases. Most patients with gastrinoma present with complaints of abdominal pain. During the secretin stimulation test, a baseline blood level is drawn. Then secretin 2 cu/kg is injected intravenously. Blood samples are drawn at intervals of 2, 5, 10, 15, and 30 minutes. In patients with gastrinoma, peak serum levels occur at 2 to 5 minutes and are normal again at 15 minutes.

EQUIPMENT

- 20-gauge angiocatheter or larger and heparin lock
- Six red-topped tubes for blood collection
- Tourniquet
- Container filled with ice (10-oz styrofoam cup)
- Vials of secretin (enough for 2 cu/kg of body weight)
- Vials of injectable saline to reconstitute secretin
- Seven 10-cc syringes (if a Vacutainer [Becton, Dickinson & Co] is used, only one 10-cc syringe is required)
- Watch or timer
- Alcohol wipes and 2x2 gauze pads with tape

NURSING IMPLICATIONS

PREPROCEDURE

- Prior to scheduling, a baseline gastrin level should be obtained.
- The patient should have NPO after midnight prior to the test.
- Discontinue PPIs and H2 blockers 72 hours prior to testing.
- Obtain a brief medical history along with allergies and medications.

General GI

Chapter 6

INTRAPROCEDURE

- The patient may sit in a chair or lie supine depending upon his or her preference.
- An IV line is placed with a 20-g angiocatheter or larger and a heparin lock placed onto the angiocatheter. This facilitates access for blood drawing. There is no need to use heparin in between the blood draws, flushing with saline is sufficient to keep the line patent.
- Apply the tourniquet for each blood draw and remove it in between blood draws.
- Draw a baseline blood level, and then inject secretin 2 cu/kg slowly over 1 to 2 minutes.
- If the patient has any untoward reaction to the secretin, stop the test and call the physician immediately. Reactions to secretin are very rare, but it has been reported that a rash or hives may occur at the injection site.
- Blood samples should be drawn at intervals of 2, 5, 10, 15, and 30 minutes.
- All vials of collected blood should be kept on ice until delivery to the appropriate laboratory for analysis.

POSTPROCEDURE

- After the test is complete, the IV line should be removed and the patient may be discharged.
- The patient should be instructed to call his or her physician if the injection site becomes red or swollen.

Appendix 1

PATIENT PREPARATION FOR ENDOSCOPIC PROCEDURES

UPPER ENDOSCOPIC PROCEDURES

- The patient should have nothing by mouth for at least 8 hours prior to the procedure.
- If the procedure entails dilation, cutting, biopsy of tissue, or the patient has a known coagulopathy, coagulation studies should be available and the patient should be advised, on the discretion of the physician, to refrain from taking aspirin, ibuprofen, or anticoagulants for 1 week prior to the procedure.
- If ERCP with sphincterotomy or PEG placement is performed, the patient should receive prophylactic antibiotics 1 hour prior to the procedure.
- Antibiotic prophylaxis is dependent upon the procedure to be performed and the discretion of the physician: for patients with prosthetic valves, history of endocarditis, pulmonary shunts, synthetic vascular grafts, mitral valve prolapse with insufficiency, cardiomoathy, congenital cardiac anomalies, cirrhosis and ascites, and those who are immunocompromised (see Table 6-2 in Chapter 6).

LOWER ENDOSCOPIC PROCEDURES

- Bowel preparation may be accomplished by using several different methods or a combination of methods:
  - ▷ Lavage method: An electrolyte lavage solution (4 L) is given at the rate of 1 to 2 L per hour after a short period of dietary restriction (light nonfibrous lunch and clear liquid supper). If the

patient cannot tolerate large amounts of oral fluid, a nasogastric tube may be inserted and the fluid poured through it. No carbohydrate-containing food or fluid should be ingested prior to or with the lavage fluid to prevent excessive sodium absorption. The solutions will not add to the circulating blood volume if used correctly and should be safe in those patients with congestive heart failure, renal impairment, or who might be subject to enhanced absorption of phosphate or sodium.

▷ Enema method: Enema until clear in combination with clear liquids or other residue-free diets for 24 to 48 hours. The enemas may be preceded by an oral cathartic such as citrate of magnesia. The drawbacks to this method are that it demands considerable time and can cause dehydration and/or hypovo- lemia if not balanced by adequate oral or intravenous intake, especially in the elderly or in those with cardiopulmonary or renal disease. In debilitated patients or those with partially obstructing colonic lesions, inflammatory bowel disease, or massive lower GI bleed, this method may be impractical and dangerous.

▷ Fleet enemas in combination with citrate of magnesia are used for flexible sigmoidoscopy. If the patient has been on clear liquids, Fleet enemas alone may be sufficient.

▷ Oral saline cathartics (Fleet phosphosoda; Johnson & Johnson Merck) in combination with suppositories (Dulcolax; Boehringer Ingelheim) and/or Fleet enemas may be used as an alternative to oral lavage and tap water enemas. This method may be more palatable than the oral lavage method because it requires ingestion of much less fluid. Health care professionals should be made aware if their patients are on a low salt diet, use diuretics for high blood pressure, have heart problems or seizures, have a history of kidney problems, or are pregnant or nursing.

• The patient should have nothing by mouth except water until just before the procedure unless general anesthesia is being used, in which case he or she should have nothing by mouth 8 hours prior to the procedure.

Appendices

Appendix 2

DISCHARGE INSTRUCTIONS FOR ENDOSCOPIC PROCEDURES

Esophagogastroduodenoscopy discharge instructions should include the following:

- Type of procedure and date performed.
- Name and phone number of the physician who performed the procedure.
- Contact phone number in case of emergency.
- Instructions for follow-up appointments or phone calls.
- If the patient develops severe epigastric pain, vomits blood, has a temperature of 101°F or higher, or becomes lightheaded or dizzy, the physician should be notified or the patient should be instructed to go to the nearest emergency room.
- No alcohol or tranquilizers should be consumed for 24 hours unless the physician states otherwise.
- Light diet progressing to regular diet should be followed by the patient as tolerated unless the physician specifies differently.
- If the patient has a sore throat after the procedure, he or she may be instructed to use throat lozenges or gargle with warm salt water for relief.
- If the intravenous site becomes painful, red, or swollen, the patient should contact his or her physician.
- No driving or strenuous activity should take place for 24 hours.

- The patient should be in the company of another person for at least 24 hours.
- The patient should be advised to avoid the use of aspirin or NSAIDs for several days after polyp removal, as directed by the physician.
- The instructions should be completed in duplicate and signed and dated by the patient or responsible party and the nurse.

Colonoscopy discharge instructions should include the following:
- Type of procedure and date performed.
- Name and phone number of the physician who performed the procedure.
- Contact phone number in case of emergency.
- Instructions for follow-up appointments or phone calls.
- If the patient develops severe lower abdominal pain, distention, or rectal bleeding (a toilet bowl full of blood and clots), develops a temperature of 101°F or higher, or becomes lightheaded or dizzy, the physician should be notified or the patient should be instructed to go to the nearest emergency room.
- No alcohol or tranquilizers should be consumed for 24 hours unless the physician states otherwise.
- Light progressing to regular diet should be followed as tolerated by the patient unless a polyp is removed, in which case a low-fiber diet is suggested for 24 hours to prevent mechanical abrasion to the polypectomy site.
- The patient may expect to be distended and bloated for the remainder of the day due to the insufflation of air into the bowel.
- Contact the physician if the intravenous site becomes red, swollen, or painful.
- No driving or strenuous activity should take place for 24 hours.
- The patient should be in the company of another person for at least 24 hours.
- The patient should be advised to avoid the use of aspirin or NSAIDs for several days after polyp removal, as directed by the physician.
- The instructions should be completed in duplicate and signed and dated by the patient or responsible party and the nurse.

Sigmoidoscopy discharge instructions should include the following:
- Type of procedure and date performed.
- Name and phone number of the physician who performed the procedure.
- Contact phone number in case of emergency.
- Instructions for follow-up appointments or phone calls.

Discharge Instructions for Endoscopic Procedures

- If the patient develops severe lower abdominal pain, distention, or rectal bleeding (a toilet bowl full of blood and clots), develops a temperature of 101°F or higher, or becomes lightheaded or dizzy, the physician must be notified or the patient should be instructed to go to the nearest emergency room.
- No alcohol, tranquilizers, or driving for 24 hours unless the physician states otherwise (only if sedation is used).
- The patient may expect to be distended and bloated for the rest of the day due to the insufflation of air into the bowel.
- The patient should be advised to avoid the use of aspirin or NSAIDs for several days after polyp removal, as directed by the physician.
- The instructions should be completed in duplicate and signed and dated by the patient or responsible party and the nurse.

ERCP discharge instructions should include the following:
- Type of procedure and date performed.
- Name and phone number of the physician who performed the procedure.
- Contact phone number in case of emergency.
- Instructions for follow-up appointments or phone calls.
- If the patient develops severe epigastric pain and vomiting, vomits blood, has a temperature of 101°F or higher, becomes lightheaded or dizzy, or becomes jaundiced, the physician should be notified or the patient should be instructed to go to the nearest emergency room.
- No alcohol or tranquilizers should be consumed for 24 hours unless the physician states otherwise.
- Light diet progressing to regular diet should be followed as tolerated by the patient unless the physician specifies otherwise. If a sphincterotomy is performed, the patient should have nothing by mouth with the exception of ice chips for the remainder of the day, progressing to a liquid diet as tolerated.
- If the patient has a sore throat after the procedure, he or she may be instructed to use throat lozenges or gargle with warm salt water for relief.
- If the intravenous site becomes painful, red, or swollen, the patient should contact his or her physician.
- No driving or strenuous activity for 24 hours. The patient should be in the company of another person for at least 24 hours.
- The patient should be advised to avoid the use of aspirin or NSAIDs for several days after polyp removal, as directed by the physician.

Appendices

Appendix 2

- The instructions should be completed in duplicate and signed and dated by the patient or responsible party and the nurse.

  Mini-Lap discharge instructions should include the following:
- Type of procedure and date performed.
- Name and phone number of the physician who performed the procedure.
- Contact phone number in case of emergency.
- Instructions for follow-up appointments or phone calls.
- Patient should not drive, operate heavy machinery, or sign legal documents after the administration of moderate sedation for at least 24 hours and should be in the company of another person for 24 hours.
- Patient should be instructed to not lift anything heavy for 48 hours.
- Diet may be as tolerated, avoiding foods that normally cause the patient to have more gas.
- No tub baths for one week, showers are allowed.
- No blood thinners, NSAIDS, or aspirin for 24 hours.
- Contact the physician if any of the following occur:
  - ▷ Redness, soreness, or purulent drainage from IV site
  - ▷ An increase in abdominal pain and/or girth
  - ▷ Weakness, dizziness, or lightheadedness
  - ▷ Increase of bloody drainage from puncture site
  - ▷ Nausea, vomiting, or fever

Appendix 3

MANUFACTURERS OF ENDOSCOPIC EQUIPMENT AND PHONE NUMBERS

The following is a brief list of manufacturers of endoscopic equipment and accessories. A complete list may be found in the Society of Gastroenterology Nurses and Associate's Buyer's Guide and Pharmaceutical Reference.

Boston Scientific Corporation
Microvasive Endoscopy
Phone: (800) 225-3226
Web site: www.bostonscientific.com

Fujinon Inc
Phone: (800) 385-4666, ext 320
Web site: www.fujinon.com

Medovations
Phone: (800) 558-6408
Web site: www.medovations.com
Email: medo@medovations.com

MedTronics Functional Diagnostics
Phone: (800) 227-3191
Web site: www.medtronic.com
Email: john.gifford@medtronic.com

Appendix 3

Olympus America Inc
Phone: (800) 645-8160
Web site: www.olympus.com

Pentax Precision Instrument Corp
Phone: (800) 431-5880
Web site: www.pentaxmedical.com

US Endoscopy Group
Phone: (800) 769-8226
Web site: www.usendoscopy.com
Email: info@usendoscopy.com

Welch Allyn Protocol
Phone: (800) 289-2500
Web site: www.welchallyn.com

Wilson Cook Medical Inc
Phone: (800) 245-4717
Web site: www.cookgroup.com

Appendix 4

List of Relevant Web Resources

American Society for Gastrointestinal Endoscopy
www.asge.org

Bard Medical Division
www.bardmedical.com

The DAVE Project
www.erbe-med.com

Ethicon Endo-Surgery, Inc.
www.inscope.com

Fleet Phosphosoda
www.phosphosoda.com

Given Imaging
http://givenimaging.com

Hemorrhoid Relief Center
www.seekrelief.com

Johns Hopkins Gastroenterology and Hepatology Resource Center
www.hopkins-gi.org

Appendix 4

Medtronic
www.medtronic.com

MUSC Pharmacy Services
www.musc.edu/pharmacy-services/medusepol/SEDATION.pdf

National Institutes of Diabetes, Digestive, and Kidney Diseases
www.niddk.nih.gov/health/health.htm

National Library of Medicine Pub Med
www.ncbi.nlm.nih.gov/PubMed/

NDO Surgical
www.ndosurgical.com

OSHA
www.osha.gov

RXmed
www.rxmed.com

The Society of Gastroenterology Nurses and Associates
www.sgna.org

UpToDate
www.uptodate.com

Wikipedia
http://en.wikipedia.org

FINANCIAL DISCLOSURES

Mr. Gerard Aguila has no financial or proprietary interest in the materials presented herein.

Dr. Stuart K. Amateau has no financial or proprietary interest in the materials presented herein.

Dr. Rukshana Cader has no financial or proprietary interest in the materials presented herein.

Dr. Marcia Irene Canto was a consultant for Pentax Medical Corporation (research grant 2009-2012).

Dr. Victor Chedid has no financial or proprietary interest in the materials presented herein.

Dr. John Clarke has no financial or proprietary interest in the materials presented herein.

Dr. Sameer Dhalla has no financial or proprietary interest in the materials presented herein.

Ms. Rosa Fusco has no financial or proprietary interest in the materials presented herein.

Financial Disclosures

Dr. Eduardo Gonzalez-Velez has no financial or proprietary interest in the materials presented herein.

Ms. Claudia Guilbeau-Brand has no financial or proprietary interest in the materials presented herein.

Dr. Christina Ha has no financial or proprietary interest in the materials presented herein.

Dr. Anthony N. Kalloo has not disclosed any relevant financial relationships.

Dr. Mouen A. Khashab has not disclosed any relevant financial relationships.

Dr. Anne Marie Lennon has not disclosed any relevant financial relationships.

Dr. Zhiping Li is a consultant for Boston Scientific.

Ms. Libbie L. Monroe has not disclosed any relevant financial relationships.

Dr. Lisette Musaib-Ali has no financial or proprietary interest in the materials presented herein.

Dr. Patrick I. Okolo III has not disclosed any relevant financial relationships.

Ms. Toshunia F. Robinson has no financial or proprietary interest in the materials presented herein.

Dr. Reem Sharaiha has no financial or proprietary interest in the materials presented herein.

Dr. Eun Ji Shin has no financial or proprietary interest in the materials presented herein.

Dr. Vikesh K. Singh is a consultant for AbbVie, Sanatarus, and D-Pharm.

Dr. Ellen Stein has no financial or proprietary interest in the materials presented herein.

Dr. David W. Victor III has no financial or proprietary interest in the materials presented herein.

Ms. Janet Yoder has no financial or proprietary interest in the materials presented herein.

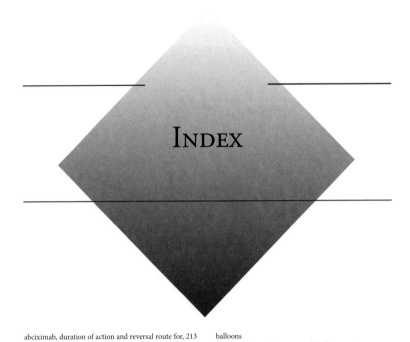

INDEX

Index

Index

Index

Index